Self-Assessment Color Review

Small Animal Ophthalmology

T0273339

Don A Samuel.

MS, PhD
Professor of Histology and Ophthalmology
Department of Small Animal Clinical Sciences
College of Veterinary Medicine
University of Florida, Gainesville, Florida, USA

Dennis E Brooks

DVM, PhD, Diplomate ACVO
Professor of Ophthalmology
Department of Small Animal Clinical Sciences
College of Veterinary Medicine
University of Florida, Gainesville, Florida, USA

MANSON PUBLISHING/THE VETERINARY PRESS

Dedication

We dedicate this work to our loved ones, who supported us during the process of its development. We especially dedicate it to our mothers, Laura Katrina Samuelson and Betty Jane Brooks, who both passed on during that time.

Acknowledgements

The creation of this book is a testament, in part, to the successful ophthalmology program that was developed by Kirk N Gelatt well over 30 years ago at the University of Florida. We, both, have been very fortunate to have been mentored by Kirk and to have worked by his side along with many faculty, residents, and graduate students, who have joined this program and been a part of our ever growing ophthalmology family. Special thanks are extended to Pat Lewis, who prepared much of the histology used in the book, and to Ashley Beattie and Suzanna Lewis for their reviewing and editing of this text.

CRC Press
Taylor & Francis Group
6000 Broken Sound Parkway NW, Suite 300
Boca Raton, FL 33487-2742

© 2011 by Taylor & Francis Group, LLC
CRC Press is an imprint of Taylor & Francis Group, an Informa business

No claim to original U.S. Government works

Printed on acid-free paper
Version Date: 20150804

International Standard Book Number-13: 978-1-84076-145-0 (Paperback)

Visit the Taylor & Francis Web site at
http://www.taylorandfrancis.com

and the CRC Press Web site at
http://www.crcpress.com

Preface

We have tried to create a book that provides a general review of small animal ophthalmology in a case-based manner. To that end we have illustrated several examples for each of the more frequent ophthalmic conditions of dogs and cats that are commonly presented to general veterinary practitioners. The differential diagnoses, examination techniques, and therapies for these ocular conditions are discussed within specific cases as well as separately. While ophthalmic problems relate to dogs and cats in similar and sometimes identical ways, there are a number of instances where this does not occur. For that reason, we have distinguished the canine cases from the feline ones in our listing of the 'Classification of cases'. For more in-depth information on differential diagnoses, examination techniques, and therapies offered in our work we encourage the reader to refer to the latest edition of Kirk Gelatt's *Veterinary Ophthalmology* (see Suggested Further Reading List).

Don A Samuelson
Dennis E Brooks

Contributors

Kathleen P Barrie DVM, Diplomate ACVO
Gil Ben-Shlomo DVM, PhD
Sarah E Blackwood DVM
Dennis E Brooks DVM, PhD, Diplomate ACVO
Catherine M Nunnery DVM, Diplomate ACVO
Caryn E Plummer DVM, Diplomate ACVO
Don A Samuelson MS, PhD
Avery A Woodworth DVM

Department of Small Animal Clinical Sciences, College of Veterinary Medicine
University of Florida, Gainesville, Florida, USA

Abbreviations

CT	computed tomography
DNA	deoxyribonucleic acid
EDTA	ethylenediamine tetra-acetic acid
MRI	magnetic resonance imaging
NSAID	nonsteroidal anti-inflammatory drug
PCR	polymer chain reaction
RNA	ribonucleic acid

Suggested further reading

Gelatt KN (2007) (ed) *Veterinary Ophthalmology*, 4th edn. Blackwell Publishing, Ames.

Maggs DJ, Miller PE, Ofri R (2008) (eds) *Slatter's Fundamentals of Veterinary Ophthalmology*, 4th edn. Saunders Elsevier, St Louis.

Martin CL (2005) *Ophthalmic Disease in Veterinary Medicine*, revised and updated edn 2010. Manson, London.

Miller PE (Consulting Editor), Tilley LP (Co-Editor), Smith FWK (Co-Editor) (2005) *The 5-Minute Veterinary Consult Canine and Feline Specialty Handbook: Ophthalmology*. Wiley-Blackwell, Hoboken.

Stades FC, Wyman M, Boeve MH *et al.* (2007) *Ophthalmology for the Veterinary Practitioner*, 2nd revised and expanded edn. Schlütersche, Hanover.

Classification of cases

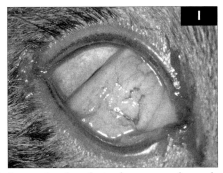

1 A nine-year-old domestic shorthaired cat was brought to the clinic for a complaint of the cat's left nictitating membrane. The third eyelid conjunctiva of this cat exhibited protrusion, chemosis, and hyperemia (1). Rose bengal stain has been applied to the eye.
i. What does rose bengal stain evaluate?
ii. What are the differential diagnoses for the conjunctivitis in this cat?

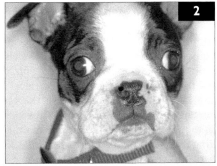

2 This 12-week-old Boston Terrier was presented for a puppy wellness examination. The owners explained that they were able to acquire the puppy for free because she had 'funny eyes' (2). They wanted to know what was wrong with the puppy's eyes.
i. What do you tell the owners?
ii. Does this condition affect vision?
iii. What can be done to resolve the condition in this puppy?

1 i. Tear film stability. The inner mucin layer of the tear film normally blocks staining of the surface epithelial cells and stroma. If the mucin layer is absent, rose bengal staining occurs. While it stains living cells, dead and degenerating cells, and mucus, this stain may have a dose-dependent ability to react with normal corneal and conjunctival epithelial cells. Rose bengal (dichloro-tetra-iodo-fluorescein) is available in solution form or impregnated paper strip. A lower concentration (0.5%) is often used, as higher concentrations (1.0% and greater) can be irritating.
ii. Herpesvirus, *Chlamydophila*, *Mycoplasma*, and bacterial infection. Conjunctivitis often accompanies viral respiratory diseases in cats. Herpesvirus is the major cause of respiratory disease with conjunctivitis in cats. Cats with chronic conjunctivitis may also be feline immunodeficiency virus positive. Often, more than one cat in a multi-cat household will be affected. Chemical and mechanical irritants may also cause conjunctivitis. Foreign bodies are frequently incriminated. Plant, upholstery, and carpet irritants may cause chemosis and conjunctivitis in cats. Household cleaners and soaps have been suspected as causes of conjunctivitis in cats. Lack of tear production is also a cause of conjunctivitis in cats. Other less common causes include hypersensitivity to topical ophthalmic preparations, parasites, and mycotic infections.

2 i. This puppy has congenital strabismus. Strabismus refers to a deviation in alignment of one globe in relation to the other globe. It may be constant or intermittent. The two eyes may be crossed (esotropia), out-turned (exotropia) as in this puppy, deviated up vertically (hyperopia), or deviated down vertically (hypotropia).
ii. Binocular vision is an acquired reflex that normally develops early in life. The development of binocular vision requires both eyes to have visual capability and to be properly aligned. Similar retinal images must project onto corresponding retinal areas of both eyes during the period of binocular vision development. Puppies with congenital or early-onset strabismus do not receive the essential visual retinal stimulation for development of binocular vision and thus lack true stereopsis. The two eyes fail to focus on the same image point, and the brain ignores the input from the deviated eye, resulting in a form of vision loss termed amblyopia.
iii. Surgical correction of the strabismus by rectus muscle transposition can be performed. Muscles can be weakened by moving the muscle insertion posteriorly or strengthened by shortening the muscle or advancing the insertion site anteriorly; alternatively, muscle insertions can be transposed to different locations in order to alter the functional pull of the muscles. Nothing but observation was done in this puppy and the strabismus self-corrected.

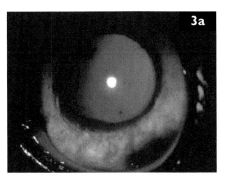

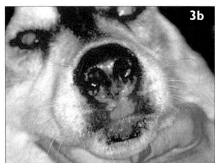

3 A seven-year-old female Husky is presented with a two-day history of blindness. Over the past month her iris color had changed from blue to brown (due to uveitis) (3a). She also has nasal depigmentation (3b) and retinal scarring (3c).

i. What is the most likely diagnosis?

ii. What breeds of dog are predisposed to this condition?

iii. What are the treatment options?

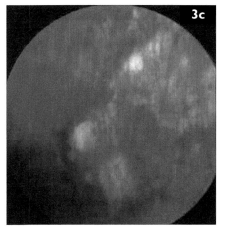

4 The owner of a seven-year-old Norwegian Forest cat had recently noticed a change in the color of her cat's right eye (4). The irides of both eyes had been normally a light blue in this nearly albinotic individual. The iris of the right eye, however, had changed during the past week to a greenish-orange. The distinctly pigmented margin around the pupil had faded considerably. What are the two main differential diagnoses of iris color change?

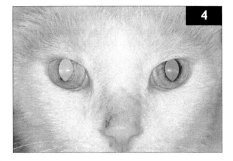

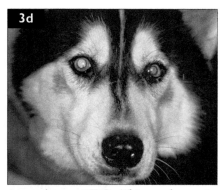

3 i. Uveodermatologic syndrome (UDS). This syndrome in the dog is similar to Vogt–Koyanagi–Harada (VKH) syndrome in humans. This immune-mediated disease against melanin is characterized by severe, bilateral panuveitis and hypotony, with secondary cataracts, glaucoma, retinal detachments, and blindness. Iris and retinal depigmentation, and poliosis/vitiligo of the face and muzzle are often noticed. Diagnosis is made from clinical lesions and breed of dog. A skin biopsy can help to confirm the condition.

ii. Originally described in the Akita, UDS has also been diagnosed in the Australian Shepherd Dog, Beagle, Brazilian Fila, Chow Chow, Dachshund, Golden Retriever, Irish Setter, Old English Sheepdog, Saint Bernard, Samoyed, Shetland Sheepdog, and Siberian Husky.

iii. The initial therapy for this condition is immunosuppressive doses of oral prednisone plus azathioprine or cyclophosphamide. After five weeks tapering, oral prednisone can begin. Most dogs require a low dose of both azathioprine and prednisone to control the disease. Topical anti-inflammatories and atropine are used to treat the uveitis (see case **12**). The eye is carefully monitored for development of secondary glaucoma. In this case the nose repigmented and the uveitis quieted following therapy (**3d**).

4 Anterior uveitis and intraocular neoplasia. Eyes with anterior uveitis may also exhibit ocular hypotony, aqueous flare, miosis, chemosis, hypopyon, keratic precipitates, and/or synechiae formation. A complete physical and ocular examination is important in order to provide diagnostic clues to the etiology of the inflammation. Intraocular melanomas and lymphoma are common in the cat and may also cause iris color change.

5 A nine-year-old spayed female dog was presented with this unilateral eye problem (**5a**).
i. Describe the clinical signs.
ii. What is your diagnosis?
iii. What are the possible causes?

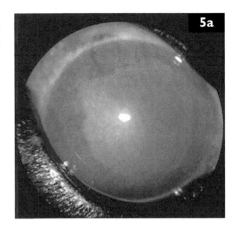

6 This nine-year-old Labrador Retriever was presented because of difficulty eating and an enlarged left eye (**6a**). There was epiphora and redness associated with the eye, and a corneal ulcer was present. The right eye appeared normal. A depigmented mass was present behind the last molar tooth of the exophthalmic side (**6b**).
i. What are the differential diagnoses?
ii. You discover that there is also a mass in the caudal aspect of the hard palate. What is the most likely diagnosis?
iii. How would you treat this condition?
iv. What is the likely prognosis?

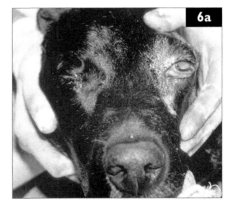

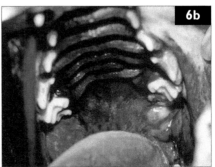

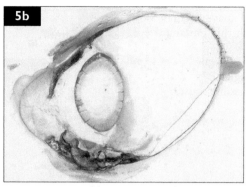

5 i. There is moderate conjunctival hyperemia with corneal vascularization at the whole corneal circumference (360°). Diffuse, severe corneal edema is noticed, but a dark mass can still be observed obliterating the anterior chamber. The Schirmer tear test is normal, there is no dazzle reflex or consensual light reflex, and the cornea is fluorescein negative.

ii. These clinical signs are consistent with glaucoma, which was confirmed by tonometry (intraocular pressure of 35 mmHg). Ocular ultrasonography revealed a mass in the anterior chamber attached to the iris. This mass was suspected to be a uveal melanoma, as this is the most common primary intraocular neoplasm in dogs. The eye was enucleated and histopathology confirmed the diagnosis (5b).

iii. Uveal melanomas in dogs are usually unilateral, rarely metastatic, destructive to the eye, and most often arise from the anterior uvea. Glaucoma may develop secondary to tumor-induced uveitis and neoplastic obliteration of the iridocorneal angle.

6 i. Orbital abscess, myosarcoma of the extraocular muscles, and orbital neoplasia (see cases 9, 146, 223).

ii. In this instance, an orbital tumor that has invaded the oral cavity. Ultrasound and CT/MRI are indicated. A biopsy revealed a fibrosarcoma.

iii. The orbit was exenterated in order to try to save the dog's life.

iv. Poor, as orbital tumors are generally malignant.

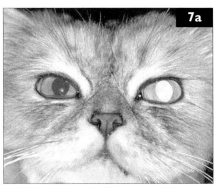
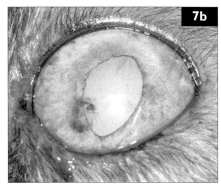

7 This adult male Norwegian Forest cat was brought to the clinic because he had been squinting in both eyes (7a, b).
i. Describe the clinical examination findings represented here.
ii. List other clinical findings that may also be present in a cat with bilateral uveitis.
iii. What are some of the more frequent causes of anterior uveitis in the cat?

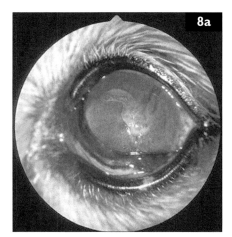
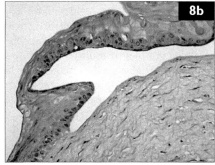

8 A 12-year-old mixed breed dog is presented with a three-week history of blepharospasm, epiphora, and a red eye with a partially opaque cornea (8a, b).
i. Describe the lesion. What is your most likely diagnosis?
ii. What breeds of dogs are prone to this condition?
iii. What is the pathology of this condition?
iv. What are the treatment options?

7 i. Hyphema is noted in the right eye. There is a focal area of fibrin mixed with red blood cells at the seven to eight o'clock position of the pupil margin in the left eye. The pupils are of similar size in both eyes. This cat has bilateral uveitis.

ii. Blepharospasm, conjunctival hyperemia, aqueous flare, hypopyon, keratic precipitates, iridal hyperemia, miosis, iris color change, decreased intraocular pressure, and decreased vision. Synechiae, cataract, lens subluxation or luxation, chorioretinitis, and secondary glaucoma may also be noted in uveitic eyes.

iii. Some of the more frequent causes of uveitis in the cat are lymphocytic-plasmacytic uveitis, feline infectious peritonitis virus, feline immunonodeficiency virus, herpesvirus, feline leukemia-associated lymphosarcoma, trauma, and lens-induced uveitis.

8 i. There is moderate conjunctival hyperemia, mild diffuse corneal edema, corneal vascularization into the central cornea (8a), and a superficial ulcer with a loose lip of epithelium at the dorsal ulcer margin (8b). The loose epithelial lip in a chronic superficial ulcer suggests this is a Boxer or indolent ulcer.

ii. Boxer, Corgi, Pekingese, and Lhasa Apso, but refractory ulcers have been documented in more than 24 breeds.

iii. Indolent corneal ulcers have been shown to have fewer hemidesmosomes and other abnormalities in the corneal epithelial basement membrane, such that the epithelium adheres to the stroma poorly. There are focal areas of epithelial separation with splitting of the basement membrane, and edema with accumulation of a basement membrane-like material.

iv. (1) The first step is débridement, with topical anesthetic and dry cotton-tipped applicators, of unattached and loosely attached epithelium. (2) Superficial grid keratotomy (GK) or multiple punctate keratotomies (MPK) also speed healing. A 20 gauge needle is used to make cross hatches ('tic tac toe') through the ulcer bed, with the scratches approximately 1–2 mm apart into adjacent normal epithelium and stroma (GK), or used to make multiple superficial punctures into the anterior stroma (MPK) and adjacent 1–2 mm of epithelium. (3) Chemical removal of the epithelium can also be accomplished with diluted topical povidone–iodine or phenol. (4) Refractory ulcers are treated medically following débridement and possible keratotomy with topical broad-spectrum antibiotic solutions, a topical cycloplegic (1% atropine) as needed, a topical hyperosmotic agent (2–5% NaCl solution) to decrease edema, and topical serum to reduce tear film protease activity. A bandage soft contact lens can also help corneal epithelial attachment.

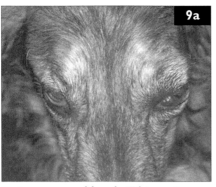
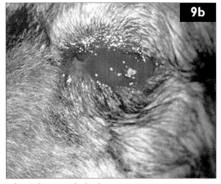

9 A two-year-old male Whippet is presented with exophthalmos, nictitans protrusion, and a muropurulent ocular discharge of his left eye (9a, b).
i. There is pain on palpation of the globe and severe blepharoconjunctivitis. What is the next step in the examination?
ii. What other diagnostic tests are indicated?
iii. What is the diagnosis, and how would you treat this condition?

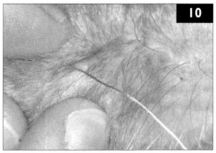

10 A diagnostic test is being performed in this adult cat (10).
i. What diagnostic test is being performed?
ii. Explain how the test is performed, and why it is used.

9 i. An oral examination under general anesthesia. A soft swelling is noted behind the last molar on the affected side (**9c**).

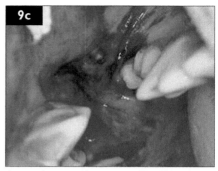

ii. Culture of the fluid from the swelling and specimens obtained for cytology. Exploration of the area is recommended after retrobulbar ultrasound or advanced imaging (CT, MRI). Ultrasound is often helpful in the diagnosis of an abscess or tumor. Advanced imaging would be helpful in determining if there is bony damage from an orbital tumor or if a foreign body is present. Ultrasound revealed a hypoechoic, 2 cm encapsulated structure in the retrobulbar space. Cytology revealed many neutrophils and bacteria.

iii. A retrobulbar abscess. Treatment is by drainage. The oral mucosa behind the last upper molar is incised and a closed hemostat slowly advanced through the pterygoid muscle. A sharp instrument should never be advanced blindly into this area of blood vessels and nerves. Damage to the maxillary artery, optic nerve, and ciliary nerves has been reported. A biopsy of the affected tissue is recommended. Irrigation of the retrobulbar area may cause increased exophthalmos and spread of the infectious organism. Systemic broad-spectrum antibiotics are indicated pending results of culture. Advanced exophthalmos may necessitate a temporary tarsorrhaphy until the swelling reduces.

10 i. The phenol red thread (PRT) test.

ii. In the PRT tear test, a 75 mm long thread is impregnated with phenol red, a pH-sensitive indicator, and used to measure tear production. A 3 mm indentation at the end of the thread is inserted into the inferior conjunctival sac for 15 seconds. The alkaline tears turn the pale yellow thread red. The mean PRT absorbance value in cats (23.0 mm/15 seconds) is approximately two-thirds the mean PRT absorbance value in dogs (34.2 ± 4.4 mm/15 seconds). Anesthesia is not necessary for the PRT tear test because the subject has little or no sensation from the thread. It is theorized that the minimal sensation and short test time give a more accurate indicator of the volume of residual tears in the inferior conjunctival sac of the eyes than the Schirmer tear test.

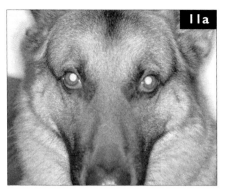
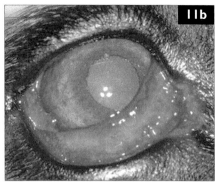

11 A three-year-old German Shepherd Dog was presented with bilateral conjunctivitis of the third eyelid (**11a, b**). The corneas appeared to be uninvolved and the dog had no previous history of ocular diseases. A cytologic sample from the conjunctiva is shown (**11c**).
i. Describe the clinical and cytologic findings.
ii. What is the diagnosis?
iii. How is this best treated?

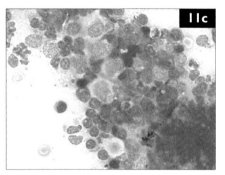

12 A cat is presented with aqueous flare, which is demonstrated by slit lamp examination (**12**).
i. What is aqueous flare?
ii. How is it treated?

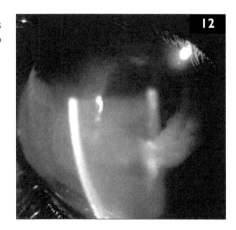

11 i. Hyperemia and thickening of the third eyelid conjunctiva. No corneal disease is present. Cytology shows plasma cells, conjunctival epithelial cells, and a few neutrophils.

ii. Plasmoma of the third eyelid, a plasma cell infiltration of the third eyelid conjunctiva that is often associated with pannus in German Shepherd Dogs. Plasmoma also has a bilateral potential in the Belgian Shepherd Dog, Borzoi, Doberman Pinscher, and English Springer Spaniel.

iii. Plasmoma is a chronic, progressive, conjunctival disorder that can be controlled in many cases by medical and/or surgical therapy, but at the present time it cannot be cured. Long-term therapy will be necessary, at a level depending on the severity of disease in the patient and the geographic location. With the exception of geographic areas of high altitude, useful vision can usually be preserved with medical therapy. Choice of drug and frequency of therapy depends on severity of lesion. Dexamethasone (0.1%) or prednisolone (1%) 1–6 times daily (to effect) is usually the first choice. As lesions regress, therapy should be reduced. Subconjunctival steroids can be given in severe cases when lesions do not respond to topical steroid or owner compliance is a problem. Cyclosporin A may also be useful in refractory cases or as maintenance therapy.

12 i. Aqueous flare occurs as protein-rich aqueous humor and cellular components accumulate within the anterior chamber after the blood–aqueous barrier has been disrupted. The interendothelial cell junctions of iris capillaries become weakened. Flare approximates the visual experience of water droplets detected by automobile headlights in fog. It is best noted in a dark room using a slit lamp biomicroscope or the small aperture of the direct ophthalmoscope in a dark room.

ii. Aqueous flare is pathognomonic for anterior uveitis. Topical anti-inflammatory therapy should be started immediately after diagnosis. Topical steroids are the treatment of choice when there is no corneal ulcer. Prednisolone acetate (1%) and dexamethasone (0.1%) (Neopolydex 0.1%) are effective topical steroid treatments for anterior uveitis. Flurbiprofen and diclofenac are topical NSAIDs that can reduce flare. Systemic NSAIDs such as carprofen have been shown to decrease flare in canine uveitis. Topical parasympatholytics agents such as atropine can also decrease flare by stabilizing the blood–aqueous barrier.

13 A young white-haired cat presents with long conjunctival hairs (**13a**).
i. Describe the clinical abnormality noted.
ii. What is the origin of this lesion?
iii. What is the treatment of choice for this particular condition?
iv. Histopathologically, what is present in this lesion?

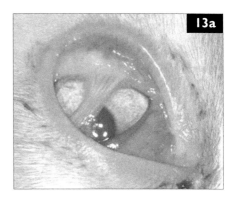

14 You are presented with a four-year-old Weimaraner dog exhibiting the condition shown (**14**). After you manipulate the mass, you determine that it is mostly associated with the nictitating membrane. You collect a dark, pigmented, thick liquid by fine-needle aspiration.
i. What is your principal diagnosis?
ii. Based on what you know about this mass, what do you tell the owner about the disease and the prognosis?
iii. What treatment will you recommend?

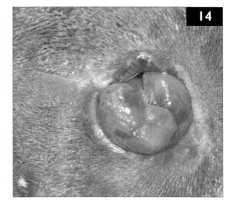

15 A six-month-old Dachshund was presented with a complaint of recurrent 'eye problems' that have occurred for the last four months (**15**). What is your diagnosis, and what is the pathophysiology of this problem?

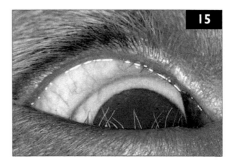

13 i. There are long hairs in association with the conjunctiva that extend or lay over the corneal surface and are beginning to cause corneal irritation. This is a conjunctival dermoid.

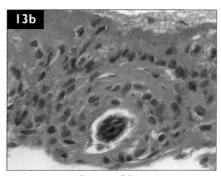

ii. A conjunctival dermoid is a benign congenital mass of ectoderm, neural crest, and mesoderm. There is abnormal invagination of the ectodermal tissue, which has resulted in a locus of differentiated dermal tissue within the conjunctiva of this cat. Dermoids may also contain cartilage and bone.

iii. Surgical removal. If removed completely, the dermoid should not return.

iv. A hair follicle is found in the dermoid (**13b**, histologic appearance of a compound ectopic hair associated with a dermoid).

14 i. Melanoma of the nictitans.

ii. Neoplasia of the third eyelid, while uncommon, is usually malignant. Recurrence after resection of malignant melanomas of the third eyelid is common. Metastasis is also common. Weimaraners may have a breed predilection for these types of tumors.

iii. The best therapy for minimizing recurrence will be resection of the mass and third eyelid and cryotherapy of the surgical site. Radiographs should be taken of the thorax to evaluate the chance of metastasis.

15 This dog is suffering from distichiasis. Distichiasis refers to single or multiple hairs arising from the meibomian duct openings at the lid margin. The meibomian glands are modified hair follicles that normally lack development of hair shafts, and distichiasis develops from undifferentiated gland tissue. Both lids can be affected and the condition is usually bilateral. Distichiasis occurs frequently in mixed breed and pure breed dogs such as the American and English Cocker Spaniel, Welsh Springer Spaniel, Cavalier King Charles Spaniel, Flat-coated Retriever, Boxer, English Bulldog, Havanese, Shetland Sheepdog, Shih Tzu, Pekingese, Tibetan Terrier and Spaniel, Dachshund, Poodle, and Jack Russell Terrier. In dogs affected with soft distichia, directed away from the cornea, the condition appears to have limited clinical significance. Stiff hairs that rub the cornea can irritate and cause lacrimation, blepharospasm, entropion, epiphora, and corneal ulcers. Distichiasis may be difficult to detect without magnifying glasses and strong, focal illumination.

16 What is the treatment of choice for the dog in **15**, and what are the risks of this treatment?

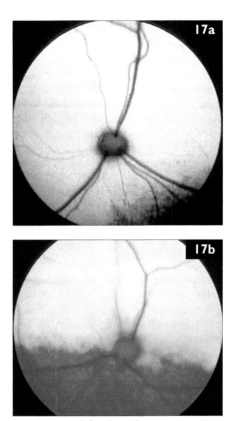

17 You are examining the normal fundus of two presenting cats.
i. List the anatomic structures shown in these direct ophthalmoscopic images of the normal feline fundus (**17a, b**).
ii. What is the term for the vascular pattern of cats?
iii. Why is the tapetal reflection of **17a** green with the nontapetum pigmented, and in **17b** the tapetal reflection is light yellow with a red coloration to the nontapetal region?

16 For permanent treatment of distichiasis the hair follicle is destroyed, removed, or redirected with surgery. The surgical methods vary from electroepilation, electrocautery, high-frequency radiohyperthermia, cryotherapy, laser ablation, partial resection of the distal tarsal plate, transpalpebral conjunctival dissection, and Hotz–Celsus lid margin repositioning; however, all have some limitations. All these methods require general anesthesia and adequate mag-

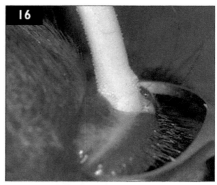

nification (5–10×) to detect the orifice of the hair and the follicle. Cryosurgery is the most popular technique (16). It is performed through the conjunctival surface directly over the follicle (3–4 mm behind the free margin of the lid). The lid margin is stabilized and everted with an eyelid clamp. A double freeze–thaw cycle using nitrous oxide specific probes destroys the follicles but spares the adjacent eyelid tissue. A -25°C 60-second freeze is followed by a brief thawing period and then a second freeze for 30 seconds. The immediate postoperative effect is considerable swelling of the cryosurgery site. Preoperative systemic NSAIDs and/or postoperative topical treatment with corticosteroid–antibiotic eye ointment are helpful. Depigmentation of the frozen areas occurs within 72 hours. Repigmentation usually takes up to six months to complete.

17 i. Tapetum, nontapetal retina, retinal vasculature, optic nerve head, and choroidal vessels. The dark ring around the optic disk is pigment in the retinal pigment epithelium and/or sclera.
ii. Holangiotic. There are three major pairs of cilioretinal arterioles and larger venules that emerge near the periphery of the optic nerve head. The retinal vessels do not anastamose on the disk surface in cats.
iii. The yellow-green hued tapetum is due to tapetal riboflavin and is the most common tapetal color in cats. The nontapetum is usually heavily pigmented. The lighter tapetum with a red nontapetum is most likely due to a very lightly pigmented cat with a light hair coat and blue irides. The redness in the nontapetum is due to the visualization of the choroidal vessels in the absence of melanocytes.

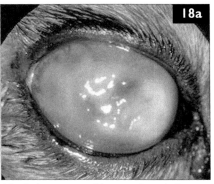
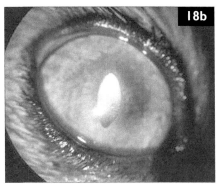

18 A four-year-old tan-colored domestic shorthaired cat presents with bilaterally afflicted corneas and conjunctivae (**18a**).
i. Describe the corneal lesions in this cat.
ii. What treatment would have been utilized to achieve the clinical result seen in **18b**?

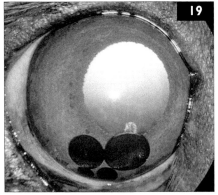

19 A six-year-old Golden Retriever is presented with dark, circular masses within the anterior chamber that the owner says have only appeared recently (**19**). The masses have distinct margins, appear to be free-floating, and can be trans-illuminated with a slit-lamp biomicroscope. There is no epiphora or evidence of ocular pain.
i. What is the diagnosis?
ii. What additional diagnostic tests could be performed to confirm your diagnosis?
iii. What is the pathophysiology of the abnormality?
iv. What treatment will you recommend?
v. If left untreated, what concerns would you have?

18 i. There is white cellular infiltrate and deep vascularization, probably the result of a viral (most likely herpesviris) infection and a secondary bacterial infection. Herpes ulcers can be linear or 'dendritic', or be large geographic ulcers as in this cat.
ii. Topical antiviral preparations and broad-spectrum antibiotics. The efficacy of antiviral medication in controlling herpesvirus conjunctivitis (without corneal involvement) remains undetermined. It can be used in severe cases, but is usually unnecessary since the condition is often self-limiting. Initial treatment includes topical 1% trifluridine or 0.1% idoxyuridine ophthalmic solution applied 3–9 times daily. The more frequent administration usually has more rapid results; however, cats can become stressed when treated this often. Vidarabine is effective topically, but can be difficult to acquire. Cidofovir (0.5%) is effective topically in cats when given BID. Systemic and/or topical alpha-2-interferon (300 U/cat PO SID; 1 drop in affected eye TID or QID) may be beneficial in cats that are refractory to other therapies. Oral famciclovir (62.5 mg/cat SID or BID for 3 weeks) is effective at reducing herpesvirus clinical signs. Lysine (250–500 mg PO BID) can reduce viral replication in latently infected cats and should be considered as a long-term therapy for cats susceptible to recurrent bouts of herpetic keratitis. If corneal ulcerations are present, concurrent treatment with a broad-spectrum topical antibiotic is advised. Stress reduction is important.

19 i. Uveal cysts (a similar example with less pigmented cysts that have yet to break away from their origin is seen in case **79**).
ii. The best diagnostic tool for differentiating a uveal cyst from a uveal tumor or neoplasia is transillumination with a slit-lamp biomicroscope. Ultrasound of the mass can also aid the diagnosis.
iii. Cysts can be acquired post trauma and/or inflammation, or they may be congenital. Congenital cysts often go unnoticed until at least a few years of age, when they become more visible. Cysts are benign and can be free-floating in the anterior chamber (see cases **27** and **79**). They can also be attached in the anterior or posterior chambers or be dislodged into the vitreous.
iv. Many cysts do not require any treatment. However, when multiple, free-floating cysts are present, they may be aspirated with a small gauge needle on a tuberculin syringe via the limbus, or deflated with a diode laser.
v. Untreated cysts have the potential to interfere with vision and/or decrease or close the iridocorneal angle, leading to secondary glaucoma. Uveal cysts in Golden Retrievers can be associated with uveitis.

20 A seven-year-old female domestic shorthaired cat is seen for her annual wellness examination, and ophthalmoscopic examination has revealed the findings shown (20).

i. Describe the clinical findings shown in this image.

ii. Between which portions of the retina is this fluid located?

iii. What changes in vision might be noted by the owner with the retinal edema noted in this cat?

iv. What may be the ultrasonographic findings in this case?

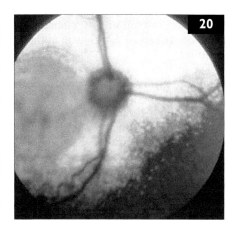

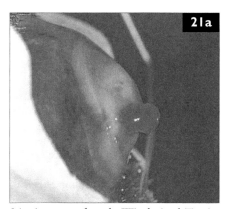

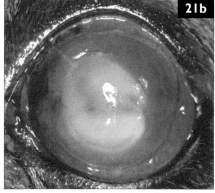

21 A young female Wirehaired Terrier was presented with an injured cornea of her left eye (21a). There was considerable pain and blepharospasm associated with this wound. The cornea had become edematous and somewhat opaque. When a fluorescein stain was applied topically to the cornea much of the region around the wound absorbed the stain (21b).

i. What is the most likely diagnosis and pathogenesis for the injured cornea in this animal?

ii. What treatments could be utilized to resolve the problem?

iii. The first image (21a) was taken after 24 hours of medical therapy. What has occurred?

20 i. There is a tan to gray, circular to ovoid lesion with distinct borders. This is a focal area of retinal detachment in the tapetum due to retinal edema and/or cellular infiltrate.

ii. The fluid and/or cells are located between the retinal pigmented epithelium and the neurosensory retina (the photoreceptor layer).

iii. The owner most likely did not notice any changes in the cat's vision. If the retina was completely detached, the owner may have noticed partial or fully dilated pupils.

iv. Subretinal fluid may be noted in a focal area of the eye.

21 i. A melting corneal ulcer. A corneal ulcer is a lesion in which epithelium and a variable amount of stroma have been lost. Corneal dissolution and liquefaction under the influence of proteases is called keratomalacia and often referred to as a 'melting cornea'. Ulcers in which proteases are active have a grayish-gelatinous, liquefied appearance around the ulcer margin, which must be distinguished from normal corneal edema. In this case the damage to the epithelium had been considerable and its role as an effective barrier against invading bacteria and other organisms had been lost. With infection, proteases and collagenases are released, mainly by neutrophils, to digest or melt the corneal collagen.

ii. (1) Broad-spectrum antibiotics are usually administered based on culture and sensitivity tests. Gentamicin, tobramycin, and/or cefazolin are recommended for initial antimicrobial therapy. (2) Autologous serum, 0.05% EDTA, and/or acetylcysteine (5%) are used topically for their collagenase and protease inhibiting properties (every 1–2 hours for the first few days, and then reduced to 3 or 4 times daily for the next 7–10 days). (3) Topical atropine therapy (1% TID) is instituted to relieve ciliary spasm and pain due to secondary anterior uveitis, and to decrease the formation of synechiae from the miotic pupil. (4) Provide corneal support of deep corneal ulcers or descemetoceles with a 360 degree, hood, island, pedicle, or bridge conjunctival flap. Amniotic membrane grafts are very good for melting ulcers. Temporary tarsorrhaphies and third eyelid flaps can be used, but are not as beneficial as conjunctival or amniotic membrane flaps.

iii. The cornea has ruptured, with the iris covered in red fibrin protruding. Surgical correction is necessary to save the eye.

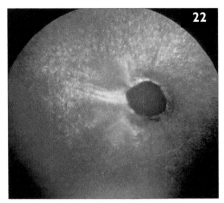

22 This one-year-old cat was presented with blindness. History revealed that it was fed a noncommercial 'vegetarian' diet.
i. Describe the ophthalmoscopic findings (**22**).
ii. What is the etiology and pathophysiology of this problem?
iii. How can it be treated?

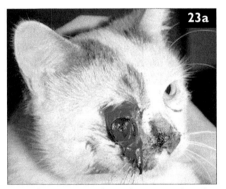
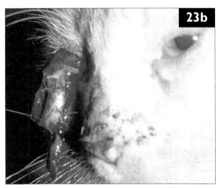

23 This young white domestic shorthaired cat is an emergency case, having been hit by a car (**23a, b**).
i. What is the most likely cause of the lesion in this cat?
ii. What is the prognosis for vision in cats that have proptosed globes (not necessarily this cat)?
iii. What simple diagnostic test can be performed in a cat with a proptosed globe to evaluate the prognosis for vision?
iv. What is the recommended treatment for this cat?

22 i. There is generalized retinal degeneration, with attenuation and loss of retinal vessels and tapetal hyperreflectivity adjacent to the optic disk at the nine o'clock position. The optic disk is very dark. The retinal degeneration was bilateral.

ii. This is a nutritional retinopathy, most likely due to a dietary deficiency in taurine. Taurine is a sulfur-containing amino acid essential to cats. Taurine has been speculated to function as a neurotransmitter and to have a protective influence on cell membranes. Ophthalmoscopic signs of taurine retinopathy become apparent between three and seven months of age, with complete retinal degeneration becoming apparent by nine months. The histopathologic appearance is one of progressive photoreceptor degeneration that is first noted in the cones and later in the rod outer segments. There are five stages of taurine retinopathy: stage 1, granularity of area centralis; stage 2, elliptical, hyperreflective lesion temporal to the optic disk; stage 3, second hyperreflective lesion nasal to optic papilla; stage 4, the two lesions coalesce; stage 5, generalized retinal degeneration with attenuation and loss of retinal vessels. Blindness occurs during stage 5. The present case is stage 5. For an example of an earlier stage see case **209**.

iii. Nutritional or taurine retinopathy is best prevented with proper diets. A dietary taurine level of 500–750 ppm has been suggested as being necessary to prevent retinal disease. The retinal effects of early taurine deficiency are only partially reversible when adequate diet is given, and irreversible in later stages. Because taurine deficiency has been linked to feline cardiomyopathy, cardiac function should be evaluated in all cats affected with these ophthalmoscopic abnormalities.

23 i. Trauma.

ii. Poor. The optic nerve in cats is very short and tolerates little stretching, especially during traumatic globe proptosis, which usually results in loss of vision. The nonproptosed normal globe must also be examined for blindness due to possible tension on the optic chiasm caused by stretching of the optic nerve from the moving injured globe.

iii. Direct and consensual pupillary light reflexes (PLRs) can be performed to evaluate the prognosis for vision. A positive PLR is a good finding.

iv. Enucleation would be the only surgical option for this cat, as the globe has collapsed and the optic nerve appears avulsed. Replacement of the globe along with medical therapy is another option if there is the possibility for return of vision. Medical therapy would consist of oral antibiotics, anti-inflammatories and analgesics, and topical antibiotics.

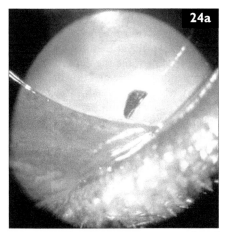

24 A five-year-old German Shepherd Dog was presented with a two-day history of blepharospasm, epiphora, and a brown spot on the eye (24a). The owner had just got back from camping with the dog.
i. What is the most likely diagnosis?
ii. What is the recommended therapy?

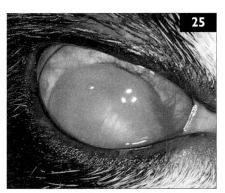

25 A nine-year-old cat is presented because of a 'change in color' of the eye (25). The owner explains that she has been managing her cat for glaucoma for the last eight months.
i. What has occurred in this cat?
ii. How does this occur?
iii. What is the treatment for this condition?

24 i. This is a corneal foreign body. The fluorescein stain can be negative if cornea has healed over the foreign body. ii. Therapy depends on how deep the foreign body has penetrated into the cornea. To determine the depth a slit lamp examination is recommended. A foreign body that is deep (24b) will be in the posterior part of the slit. Corneal foreign bodies are removed in order to limit pain, reduce the potential for infection, and prevent vascularization and scar formation. Small, superficial foreign bodies are removed with topical anesthesia and saline irrigation, cotton tip débridement, ophthalmic forceps, or a needle-shaped instrument. Deep foreign bodies should be removed under general anesthesia, and may require corneal suturing and placement of a conjunctival flap. After removal of the foreign body, a broad-spectrum topical antibiotic and atropine are administered to limit infection and control pain due to secondary uveitis.

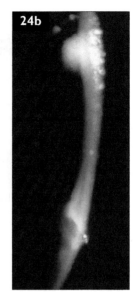

25 i. This cat has an anteriorly luxated cataractous lens. Anterior lens luxation causes an obvious loss in anterior chamber depth.
ii. Luxation of the lens in cats is most common as a sequela to chronic uveitis (see case 32) or glaucoma. The opposite scenario of glaucoma being caused by lens luxation is not as common in cats as in dogs due to the larger anterior chamber depth of cats. The anterior luxation causes the lens and corneal endothelium to be in contact, resulting in corneal endothelial damage, elevated intraocular pressure due to the lens blocking aqueous humor movement at the pupil, and often persistent uveitis. Primary lens luxation can also occur as a result of weakness in the zonular fibers.
iii. If the cause of the luxation is primary, intracapsular lens extraction is much more successful than if the luxation is secondary to uveitis. In diseased eyes with secondary luxation, the disease may complicate the surgical outcome. However, surgery is still recommended if retinal function is normal. Careful attention should be given to the treatment if uveitis or glaucoma is associated with the luxation.

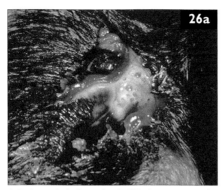
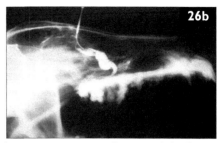

26 An adult female Collie is presented with a severe mucopurulent nasal discharge (26a). Dacryocystorhinography was performed on the patient (26b).
i. What are the clinical signs associated with dacryocystitis?
ii. What is the purpose of dacryocystorhinography?
iii. Describe how the procedure of dacryocystorhinogram is performed.
iv. How should this dog be treated?

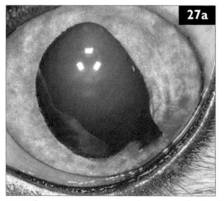
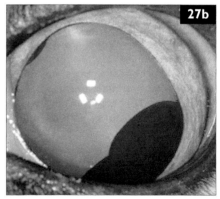

27 The owner notices a brown spherical structure at the pupil margins in a three-year-old neutered domestic shorthaired cat (27a, b).
i. What is the diagnosis?
ii. How might this condition be treated?

26 i. Clinical signs include ocular discharge, either epiphora or mucopurulent discharge, swelling in the medial periorbital area, blepharospasm, and conjunctivitis.

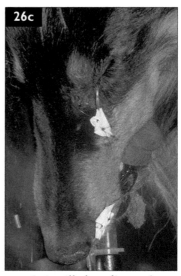

ii. To identify obstruction of the nasolacrimal duct from inflammation, infection, masses, rupture or incomplete development, deviation of the lacrimal drainage system, dilation of the lacrimal sac, and orbital and nasal osteolysis. The photo of dacryocystorhinography (26b) shows dilation of the lacrimal sac and duct in association with dacryocystitis, and duct obstruction and rupture.

iii. Dacryocystorhinography is performed under general anesthesia. Sterile saline is used to flush the nasolacrimal duct. About 0.5–1 ml of radiopaque ionic or nonionic iodinated contrast material is injected into the nasolacrimal puncta through cannulation of the duct. Once the contrast is instilled, radiographs or fluoroscopy are performed to visualize the nasolacrimal duct drainage system.

iv. The nasolacrimal duct should be cannulated with silastic tubing to allow the infection to drain and cause recannulization of the duct (26c).

27 i. A uveal cyst. Compare this case with case 53. In this case the uveal cyst is very dense and a slit lamp is needed to transilluminate it. Uveal cysts may arise from the posterior pigment epithelium of the iris or from the inner ciliary body epithelium; they can be congenital or acquired. In both this case and case 53 they are identified by their spherical shape and translucency when illuminated with intense, focal light sources, and are frequently positioned at the pupillary margins. If the uveal cyst is very dense and pigmented, high frequency ultrasound can help with the diagnosis.

ii. An argon laser can be used to rupture, coagulate, and deflate the cyst.

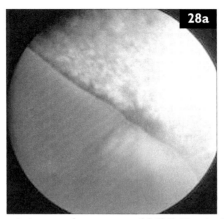

28 An ophthalmoscopic image of a ten-year-old Shih Tzu is shown (28a).
i. What is the pathology?
ii. What are the etiology and treatment?

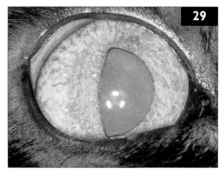

29 A five-year-old domestic shorthaired cat presents with an abnormal pupil shape (29).
i. Describe the clinical findings in this cat's right eye.
ii. Describe the neural innervations to the iris.
iii. How is it possible for this cat to have a pupil that is D-shaped?
iv. Why cannot a pupil of this shape be found in the dog?

28 i. This is a giant rhegmatogenous retinal detachment. A rhegmatogenous detachment is one that is associated with a tear or hole in the layers of the sensory or neural retina. The retinal defect allows vitreous and fluid to dissect the neuroretina from the retinal pigmented epithelium, thus exacerbating the size and significance of the lesion.

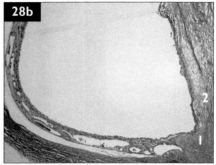

ii. Rhegmatogenous retinal detachments from retinal tears can be congenital (28b, 1 = optic nerve; 2 = retina), be associated with Collie eye anomaly, result post-cataract surgery, occur with retinal dysplasia, and result from glaucoma. Retinal tears may be focal or giant retinal detachments that involve the entire retina. Giant retinal detachments are common in breeds such as the Shih Tzu. Retinopexy can be used to try and stop the retinal detachment progress.

29 i. There are prominent iris vessels associated with the lateral and medial iris. The pupil resembles the letter 'D'.

ii. Parasympathetic nerves innervate the iris sphincter muscle and sympathetic nerves innervate the iris dilator muscle. The long ciliary nerves are branches of the nasociliary nerve that branch off the ophthalmic branch of the trigeminal nerve. They provide both sympathetic efferent and somatosensory afferent nerve fibers to the iris. These sympathetic fibers innervate the iris dilator muscle. Parasympathetic fibers in the oculomotor nerve synapse at the ciliary ganglion and then become the short ciliary nerves that innervate the iridal sphincter muscle.

iii. The cat has two short ciliary nerves from the ciliary ganglion. The malar short ciliary nerve is lateral and the nasal short ciliary nerve is medial. They each innervate their respective half of the iris sphincter muscle. Lesions to the medial aspect or nasal short ciliary nerve result in iris sphincter hemiplegia or a D-shaped pupil, as noted in this cat's right eye. A lesion to the lateral aspect or malar short ciliary nerve results in a reversed-D-shaped pupil in the right eye. Lesions in the left eye are reversed.

iv. The neural anatomy of the short ciliary nerves differs between the cat and the dog. In the dog a lesion associated with the parasympathetic innervation to the iris sphincter muscle results in dilation of the pupil equally in both the medial and lateral aspects.

30 A 14-day-old Golden Retriever puppy has just opened his eyes (30).
i. At what age do the eyelids normally open in puppies and kittens?
ii. What are the risks of premature opening of the eyelids?

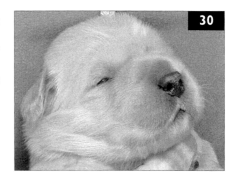

31 A three-year-old domestic long-haired cat was presented with a two-day history of blepharospasm, epiphora, and conjunctivitis. A rose bengal stain was applied to the right eye and resulted in an uptake in a linear, branching pattern in the dorsal cornea (31).
i. What is the most likely cause of such a staining pattern?
ii. What is the importance of using rose bengal stain?
iii. What is the etiology of this disease?
iv. What are the treatment options?

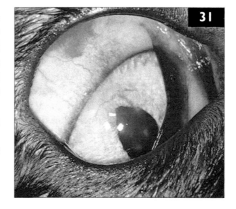

32 An adult female Siamese cat was being treated for anterior uveitis. When she was brought back for a re-examination, the present condition was noticed (32).
i. What is the diagnosis of this condition in this cat?
ii. What are possible etiologies for this condition?
iii. What are the possible treatments for this condition?

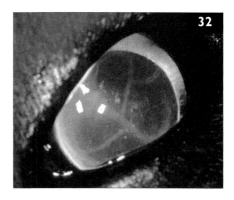

30 i. The canine and feline palpebral fissure is normally sealed during the second and third trimesters of fetal development, respectively, and opens at 10–14 days postpartum.
ii. The postpartum ankyloblepharon period is needed due to the relative immaturity of the ocular and adnexal tissue at birth. A natural or iatrogenic early opening of the palpebral fissure will usually lead to exposure keratoconjunctivitis and moderate to severe corneal ulceration. Corneal rupture is a possible complication. In cases of premature opening of the palpebral fissure, frequent administration of artificial tear ointment is necessary to protect the ocular surface. Temporary tarsorrhaphy for 10–14 days should be considered, especially if the palpebral fissure opens peripartum.

31 i. The large rose bengal uptake over the dorsal bulbar conjunctiva is due to the touch application of the rose bengal strip. The linear dendritic staining pattern of the cornea represents a herpes ulcer in this cat.
ii. Rose bengal dye evaluates the stability of the mucin layer of the tear film. If the mucin layer is abnormal, exposed superficial epithelial cells and stroma can stain magenta.
iii. A dendritic ulcer is pathognomonic for herpes keratitis in a cat. Feline herpes-virus-1 is a widespread disease with an estimated 50–97% of cats being seropositive. The dendritic lesions indicate viral movement along the superficial corneal nerves from the trigeminal ganglion.
iv. Therapy consists of topical antiviral preparations and broad-spectrum antibiotics to control secondary bacterial infections (for further details see cases **11** and **130**).

32 i. Anterior lens luxation, as determined by the visible aphakic crescent laterally.
ii. Luxation can be associated with trauma, chronic uveitis, and glaucoma. The zonules are weakened by inflammation or mechanical stretching to such an extent that they break and allow the lens to shift from its normal position.
iii. Surgical treatment for lens luxation is intracapsular lens extraction before permanent ocular changes occur. Anteriorly luxated lenses can lead to corneal endothelial damage, glaucoma, and retinal detachment if not surgically removed. Posteriorly luxated lenses can be associated with ocular discomfort and retinal detachment.

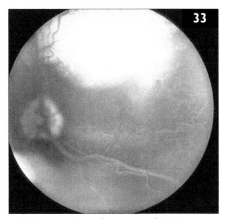

33 This retinal image (33) was taken from a male Miniature Schnauzer.
i. What condition is depicted in the retinal vessels?
ii. List some common systemic diseases that may cause this manifestation.
iii. Is the syndrome usually unilateral or bilateral?
iv. What diagnostic tests should be run if the condition is suspected?
v. What is the treatment for this eye condition?

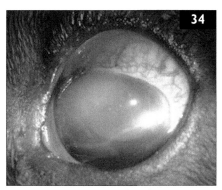

34 An eight-year-old cattle dog presents with a four-week history of a blue cornea (34).
i. Describe the ocular abnormalities.
ii. What is the cause of the Haab's striae in the central cornea?
iii. What are the treatment options for this globe condition?

33 i. Lipemia retinalis from hyperlipidemia, as seen by the pale pink retinal vasculature. Excessive plasma chylomicrons are present. This condition is more easily identified when the retinal vessels over the nontapetal retina are visualized.
ii. Lipemia retinalis and hyperlipidemia can be a primary condition in the Miniature Schnauzer. Pancreatitis, high-fat diets, postprandial, glomerulonephropathy, hypothyroidism, diabetes mellitus, hyperadrenocorticism, and renal or hepatic disease are causes of secondary hyperlipidemia.
iii. This syndrome is systemic and therefore bilateral.
iv. General blood work and fasting triglycerides and cholesterol levels are evaluated. Urinalysis, a thyroid panel, and testing for Cushing's disease should also be run if indicated.
v. Lipemia retinalis is not associated with ocular pathology. The primary disease is treated as indicated by the results of diagnostic testing. Low-fat diets should be implemented.

34 i. There is episcleral injection, mild diffuse corneal edema, Haab's striae (linear streaks of edema), dorsal lens subluxation, and the pupil is dilated.
ii. A rupture in Descemet's membrane. Uncontrolled intraocular pressure (IOP) elevation will stretch the globe and cornea to cause breaks in Descemet's membrane. Aqueous enters the area, causing regions of linear edema along the break.
iii. The clinical signs indicate that the eye is glaucomatous. Treatment options are medical and surgical (see case **81**). Multiple drug therapy decreases IOP by reducing production of aqueous humor and diminishing the resistance to aqueous humor outflow. Topical carbonic anhydrase inhibitors (e.g. dorzolamide, brinzolamide) reduce aqueous humor production. Topical beta-adrenergic antagonists (e.g. timolol, betaxolol) reduce aqueous humor production. Topical prostaglandins (e.g. latanaprost, travaprost) increase aqueous humor outflow through the uveoscleral pathway. Topical parasympathomimetic drugs (e.g. pilocarpine, demecarium bromide) act primarily to cause ciliary muscle contraction, increasing the outflow of aqueous humor. Oral carbonic anhydrase inhibitors (acetazolamide, 10–25 mg/kg PO BID; dichlorphenamide, 5–10 mg/kg PO BID; methazolamide, 5 mg/kg PO BID) reduce ciliary body production of aqueous humor. Hyperosmotics (mannitol, 1–2 g/kg IV QID; glycerol, 1–2 mg/kg PO QID) lower IOP rapidly by osmotically reducing the volume of the vitreous and are only effective for a few hours.

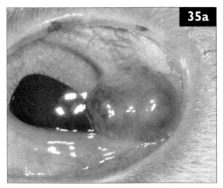

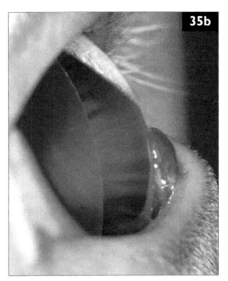

35 A seven-year-old neutered domestic shorthaired cat was presented for ophthalmic examination (35a, b).
i. What is the tan structure seen at the three o'clock position of the cornea?
ii. How would you treat it?

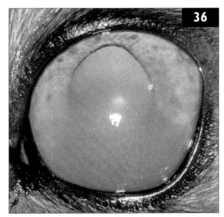

36 A 12-year-old Siamese cat is presented with a painful, slightly enlarged cloudy eye (36). There is ventral corneal edema, aqueous flare, and the iris is mottled in appearance. The intraocular pressure (IOP) is 45 mmHg.
i. What is the most likely diagnosis?
ii. What is the etiology of this condition?
iii. What therapy is recommended, and what is the prognosis for vision?

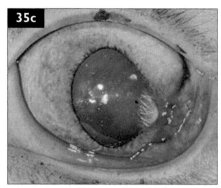

35 i. The iris, which was prolapsed due to full-thickness perforation of the cornea. This condition can develop from the progression of deep corneal ulcers or from trauma.

ii. Corneal perforations can be treated successfully with conjunctival flaps and grafts. This photo (35c), which was taken of the eye one month later, shows how well the perforation has healed.

36 i. Uveitis-induced secondary glaucoma.

ii. The anterior uveitis has caused iris swelling and blockage of the iridocorneal angle with scar tissue and inflammatory debris. The onset of clinical signs of uveitis-induced glaucoma in cats is often insidious, as cats are less likely to demonstrate the acute intense corneal edema and episcleral congestion exhibited in dogs. All ocular tissues are eventually affected by the elevated IOP.

iii. Multiple drug therapy to decrease IOP by reducing production of aqueous humor and diminishing the resistance to aqueous humor outflow. A topical beta blocker (timolol maleate, 0.5% BID) and a topical carbonic anhydrase inhibitor (1% brinzolamide or 2% dorzolamide, TID), plus topical and systemic steroids to reduce the signs of uveitis, can be beneficial in cats with glaucoma. Frequent IOP monitoring is essential. Surgery should be considered when the IOP cannot be controlled medically. Anteriorly luxated lenses should be removed in functioning eyes to relieve pupillary block and prevent corneal damage due to the lens touching the corneal endothelium. A diode laser can be used to cause ciliary body necrosis (cyclophotocoagulation) to lower IOP. Gonioimplants can shunt aqueous humor around the blocked drainage angle to lower IOP. Enucleation is indicated when vision is lost in uncontrolled glaucoma. The prognosis for vision is not good in this eye as controlling the uveitis may be difficult.

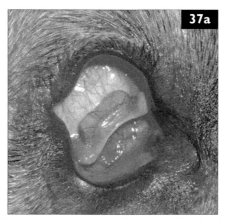

37 A one-year-old Great Dane is presented with ocular discharge, chemosis, and 'cherry eye', with folding of the nictitating membrane (37a).
i. What is the diagnosis?
ii. Discuss the pathophysiology involved in this condition.
iii. Describe two surgical corrections for this condition.

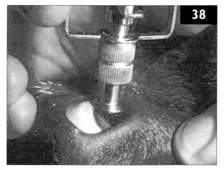

38 One method of measuring intraocular pressure (IOP) is the use of Schiotz tonometry (38).
i. What is a Schiotz tonometer?
ii. How is the device used, and what are the normal IOP readings using the Schiotz?

37 i. Everted cartilage of the nictitating membrane and idiopathic prolapse of the gland of the nictitating membrane ('cherry eye').

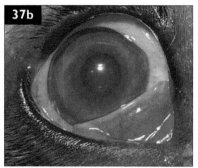

ii. The pathophysiology of 'cherry eye' is not fully known. It is thought to result from weak connective tissue attachments between the periorbital tissues and the ventral portion of the membrane. Once the gland has become exposed, it enlarges due to chronic exposure. Everted nictitans cartilage occurs due to folding of the anterior edge of the nictitating membrane, with subsequent exposure of the posterior portion. This condition is caused by faster growth of the posterior portion of the nictitans cartilage compared with the anterior component.

iii. Excision of the folded section of the cartilage is recommended for correction of everted nictitans cartilage. Two options have been described for surgical repair of a prolapsed gland: simple excision of the gland or replacement of the gland into its normal position (**37b**). The pocket technique for replacement requires the creation of a subconjunctival pocket of the nictitans conjunctiva, leaving a small opening at either end of the pocket to prevent cyst formation. The prolapsed gland is buried in the pocket. In the anchoring technique, a suture is placed through the periosteal tissue of the orbital rim in order to pull the gland back into its natural position behind the orbital rim.

38 i. It is an indentation tonometer. The routine use of Schiotz tonometry is more accurate than digital tonometry, is relatively inexpensive, and is a valuable diagnostic aid. The tonometer consists of a corneal footplate, plunger, holding bracket, recording scale, and 5.5, 7.5, 10.0, and 15.0 g weights. The low friction plunger within the corneal footplate indents the cornea proportionally to the IOP. The accuracy of Schiotz tonometry depends on the clinician and the patient. The Schiotz tonometer should not be used on corneas with deep ulcers.

ii. Measurement of IOP with the Schiotz tonometer in small animals is relatively easy. Topical anesthetic is applied to both eyes. The animal is placed in a sitting position or in lateral or dorsal recumbency. The eyelids are held open and the animal's head elevated dorsally. The tonometer is held vertically and placed on the center of the cornea just long enough for the measure to be read off the scale. The conversion table provided with the instrument is used to determine IOP.

Using a 5.5 g weight, the IOP is normal in a dog if the Schiotz scale reads between 3 and 7, and in the cat if the scale reads between 2 and 6. Readings <2–3 suggest ocular hypertension and readings >7 suggest ocular hypotension.

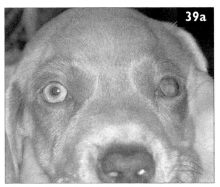
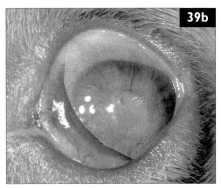

39 A 14-week-old female Weimaraner puppy was presented with a unilateral lesion associated with her left eye (39a).
i. Describe the corneal lesions in 39b.
ii. This dog suffered from neonatal ophthalmia. What are the causes and treatment for this condition?

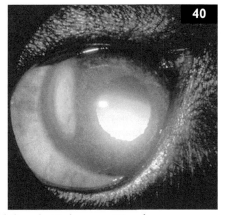

40 A three-year-old female Doberman Pinscher was presented with a corneal problem of her left eye (40).
i. Describe the clinical abnormalities observed.
ii. What systemic abnormalities can be associated with this keratopathy?
iii. What is the theory behind how the substance is deposited in the cornea?
iv. If systemic abnormalities are associated with this corneal condition, are there treatments that can be used to remove these deposits in the cornea?

39 i. The cornea is heavily vascularized 360° around the limbus, with severe, diffuse, corneal edema and fibrosis. Corneal fluorescein staining is negative in this case, indicating that a corneal ulcer is not present.

ii. Neonatal ophthalmia is an infection of the conjunctiva and/or cornea that results from premature breakdown of the palpebral fissure. This infection is usually associated with staphylococcal keratoconjunctivitis in dogs; in cats it may be caused by feline herpesvirus. Infectious organisms enter the conjunctival sac presumably via a small patent opening at the medial canthus. The first indications of neonatal ophthalmia may be a slight purulent discharge at the medial canthus and/or bulging of the eyelids due to accumulation of inflammatory debris between the lids. Symblepharon (adhesions of the conjunctiva to the cornea) may develop in some eyes with neonatal ophthalmia. Corneal perforation and iris prolapse are occasionally seen. The first step in treatment is careful opening of the palpebral fissure by manual traction, beginning at the medial canthus, and drainage of any purulent material touching the cornea. Warm compresses may help in separation of the eyelids. The conjunctival sac and cornea should be lavaged with warm saline or 1:50 povidone–iodine aqueous solution and the discharge removed. The eyes should be treated with topical, broad-spectrum antibiotics QID until the condition resolves.

40 i. The condition seen is corneal lipidosis (lipid keratopathy). There is a vertical ovoid, white to blue opacity associated with the lateral peripheral cornea. Usually there is also a clearer peripheral perilimbal zone with this condition. Corneal lipidosis is usually found with no corneal vascularization, but vascularization can occur in chronic cases.

ii. Hypothyroidism, diabetes mellitus, pancreatitis, hyperlipoproteinemia, and postprandial plasma lipid elevations can cause lipid keratopathy in dogs. These biochemical changes can be evaluated by blood tests.

iii. The theory is that the perilimbal blood vessels deposit the lipid into the cornea, or that there is in-situ lipid deposition.

iv. Dietary change to a low-fat diet may stop the deposition of further lipid or decrease the amount of deposits within the cornea. If, through serum biochemistry analysis, a disease process such as hypothyroidism or diabetes mellitus is diagnosed, treating the disease may stop the progression of lipid deposition or minimize the number of opacities within the cornea. Keratectomy to remove the lipid deposits is possible, but unless the source of the deposition is identified deposition will continue.

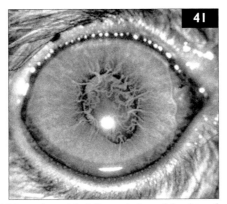

41 A four-week-old kitten has this bilateral thread-looking lesion in its eye (41).
i. What is the most likely diagnosis?
ii. Why are these structures tan to white in color?

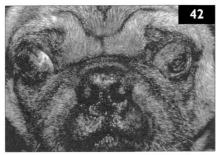

42 A five-year-old Pug was presented with bilaterally dry eyes. The anterior epithelium of the corneas and bulbar conjunctivae had become notably thickened. While neither eye had any obvious ulceration, blinking resulted in considerable pain. Initially, the eyes were red and inflamed, with some mucopurulent discharge. Cultures yielded little useful information. The dog was thought to have been exposed to some irritant or even possibly have bacterial conjunctivitis. Eventually, the condition illustrated (42) arose.
i. What are the most common etiologies of keratoconjunctivitis sicca (KCS) in dogs and cats?
ii. Describe the diagnostic procedures useful in animals with KCS.
iii. What is the most effective treatment for KCS?

41 i. Persistent pupillary membranes (PPMs). In the fetus the pupil is closed with a thin pupillary membrane (tunica vasculosa lentis) that regresses prior to birth. Sometimes, regression is not complete at birth and web-like strands are still present until 4–5 weeks of age. PPMs are rare in cats and may present in normal eyes or eyes with multiple ocular anomalies. They vary in size and shape from one individual to another (see case **248**).

ii. PPMs are generally brown or the color of the iris. They are a remnant of the tunica vasculosa lentis, a vascular structure of the fetal lens. The PPMs in this kitten are still patent and are tan to white because of increased levels of serum lipids.

42 i. Iatrogenic loss of lacrimal tissues due to surgical removal of the nictitans gland in cherry eye procedures; congenital and/or breed-related hypoplasia or aplasia of the tear-forming glands; eyelid and tarsal gland agenesis in cats. A reduction in tears can also occur from chronic, diffuse conjunctival infiltration and destruction of conjunctival goblet cells. Chronic conjunctivitis or blepharitis can affect the duct openings of the tarsal (meibomian) glands by closing and plugging the ducts, resulting in KCS. The use of topical atropine, several sulfonamides, and topical anesthetics can result in KCS. Atropine can temporarily reduce lacrimal gland secretion, so where topical atropine is used with ulcerated corneas, it is imperative to document and monitor tear production. Systematically administered sulfonamides (e.g. phenazopyridine, sulfadiazine, sulfasalazine) have a toxic and often permanent effect on the secretory cells of the lacrimal gland. A loss of lacrimal gland neural innervation due to traumatic, infectious, iatrogenic, neoplastic, and other conditions will result in lacrimal gland inactivity. Most KCS in dogs appears to be a result of an immune-mediated attack on the lacrimal gland (see case **199**). Radiation therapy can also destroy lacrimal gland tissue and cause KCS in dogs.

ii. The Schirmer tear test (STT), which can be performed either with or without the use of a topical anesthetic; fluoroscein staining of affected eye(s) to detect corneal ulcers; use of rose bengal stain to evaluate tear film stability and adherence.

iii. Most eyes treated with cyclosporin A or tacrolimus respond with increased tear production, although it may take several weeks of therapy to reach maximum STT levels.

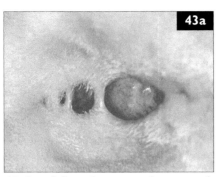

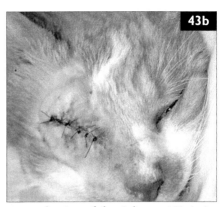

43 An adult cat is presented one month post enucleation of the right eye (43a). An orbital exenteration surgery was necessary to resolve the condition (43b).
i. Describe and define the tissue seen underneath the skin laceration.
ii. Describe two enucleation methods and how to prevent the above complication.

44 This eight-year-old male mixed breed dog has a corneal burn injury that has led to a corneal degeneration (44).
i. What is corneal degeneration?
ii. What is the hallmark clinical sign of corneal degeneration?
iii. Describe the appearance of calcium in the cornea.
iv. Describe the appearance of lipid in the cornea.
v. Why are lipid and calcium deposited within the cornea?

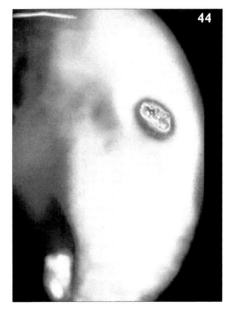

43 i. There is a pink, glistening tissue underneath the skin laceration. This appears to be conjunctiva of the nictitating membrane. The conjunctiva, lacrimal gland, and nictitating membrane should have been removed as part of the original enucleation surgery.
ii. The most commonly used enucleation technique is the subconjunctival approach. Beginning in the dorsal quadrant, the bulbar conjunctiva is incised approximately 5 mm posterior to the limbus. The conjunctiva and Tenon's capsule are bluntly dissected from the globe and the extraocular muscles are identified and transected close to their scleral insertion. Medial rotation of the globe will expose the optic nerve, which is clamped with curved hemostats and then transected behind the globe. Two to three millimeters of eyelid margins are then removed and the subcutaneous tissue closed with absorbable sutures. The eyelids are closed with simple interrupted sutures using 4-0 nonabsorbable monofilament suture material. A second technique is the transpalpebral enucleation approach in which the eyelids are sutured together in a continuous suture pattern. Two elliptical incisions, approximately 2–3 mm behind the lid margins, are joined near the medial and lateral canthus. Deep dissection will identify the bulbar conjunctiva. Forward traction of the eyelids will help with dissection of the conjunctiva until the sclera is encountered at the limbus. Further posterior dissection and removal of the globe is the same as that for the subconjunctival approach. Care should be taken not to stretch the optic nerve during enucleations.

44 i. Corneal degenerations can consist of lipid, cholesterol, or calcium, and are associated with collagen breakdown, corneal vascularization, and corneal pigmentation. The burn that had occurred in this dog has resulted in degenerative changes to the cornea.
ii. Vascularization of the cornea.
iii. Calcium appears as punctate, irregular, white, superficial or deep, shiny opacities.
iv. Lipid appears as off-white colored crystalline opacities. They can be superficial or deep in the cornea.
v. Necrotic cells release crystalline and noncrystalline lipids. Fibroblasts and keratinocytes may form lipid after inflammation or injury. Vascularization may allow for hematogenous lipid deposition. Calcium is deposited commonly in inflamed corneas because the corneal calcium levels are close to saturation and small changes in pH or temperature easily result in calcium precipitation.

45 A 15-year-old domestic short-haired cat was presented with bilateral acute blindness. Funduscopic examination of the right eye revealed the condition shown (45a).

i. Describe the lesion.

ii. What is the most likely cause of this lesion, and what would be the treatment?

iii. What is the prognosis for return of vision?

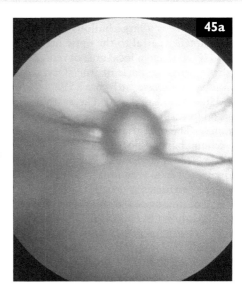

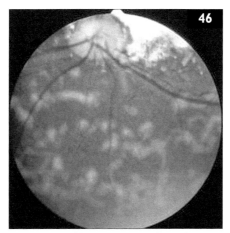

46 A three-year-old Border Collie is presented with active chorioretinitis and blindness (46). Ivermectin had been administered one day prior.

i. What is the most likely diagnosis?

ii. What is the pathogenesis of this condition?

iii. What breeds are predisposed to this condition?

iv. What is the treatment and prognosis?

45 i. There is a large bullous retinal detachment ventral to the optic nerve head (ONH) and a focal area of retinal edema dorsal (left) of the ONH. Compare this case with case **159**.

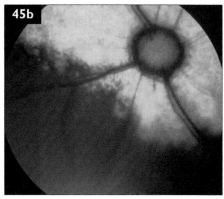

ii. High blood pressure. The systolic blood pressure in this cat was 230 mmHg. The treatment of choice was a calcium channel blocker (amlodipine, 0.625–1.25 mg per cat PO SID) to lower the blood pressure.

iii. The prognosis is dependent on the length of time since the retina detached and the ability to control the blood pressure (**45b**, vision has returned in ten days as the retina has reattached following blood pressure reduction). There is some evidence that the feline retina begins to degenerate within the first week of detachment. Retinal hemorrhages and edema can resolve with appropriate therapy.

46 i. Ivermectin-induced chorioretinitis or toxic chorioretinopathy. There are multifocal, light gray, round to linear areas in the nontapetal fundus (**46**).

ii. Ivermectin is an antiparasitic drug that activates ligand-gated chloride channels in invertebrates, paralyzing the parasite. Therapeutic levels of ivermectin do not normally reach toxic levels in the CNS of mammals due to P-glycoprotein on the vascular endothelial cells of the blood–brain barrier. The P-glycoprotein prevents a variety of molecules from entering the CNS. The P-glycoprotein is coded for by the multiple drug resistance gene (MDR-1). Animals with this mutant gene cannot prevent ivermectin from crossing the blood–brain barrier.

iii. Breeds found to carry the mutant MDR-1 allele include the Australian Shepherd Dog, Miniature Australian Shepherd Dog, Collie, English Shepherd, Long-haired Whippet, Old English Sheepdog, Shetland Sheepdog, and the Silken Windhound.

iv. The therapy is supportive care. Animals typically make a full recovery with return of vision in 2–10 days, but can take many weeks. Residual pigment disruption may be visible in the nontapetal region after recovery. Severely affected dogs may die from respiratory/cardiovascular compromise.

47 A 10-year-old spayed female cat is seen with a two-month history of a pink mass growing in the medial canthus and lower eyelid (47a).

i. What are the differentials for this mass?

ii. What are the treatment options?

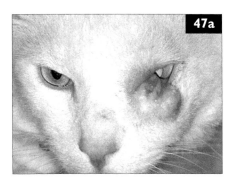

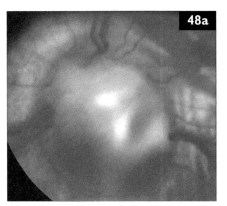

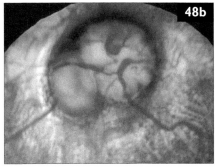

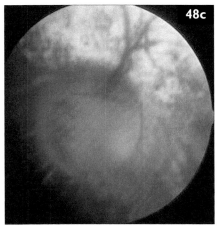

48 What is the etiology of the ocular condition found in these three images (48a–c)?

47 i. Differentials include squamous cell carcinoma (SCC), basal cell carcinoma, mast cell tumor, fibrosarcoma, papilloma, adenoma, adenocarcinoma, fibroma, neurofibroma, neurofibrosarcoma, melanoma, hemangioma, hemangiosarcoma, and myxosarcoma. The most likely possibility for a lid tumor in a white cat or a cat with nonpigmented eyelid margins is SCC, although in this instance it turned out to be myxosarcoma. Eyelid tumors in cats are less common, but generally more malignant, than those in dogs.

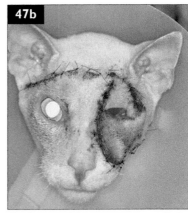

ii. The treatment options for eyelid tumors are surgical. Since the potential for malignancy is high, careful examination of the whole animal is indicated, and cytology of local lymph nodes is recommended. Surgical removal with wide-based excision and adjunctive therapy is the treatment of choice. The goal of surgery is to restore eyelid margins and prevent trichiaisis with secondary keratitis. Adjunctive therapies include cryotherapy, beta-irradiation, laser ablation, and hyperthermia. Blepharoplasty may be required when tumors are extensive. A rotational graft was used in this cat (47b). The upper lip of the mouth was rotated to create a lower eyelid with a mucous membrane margin.

48 Each of these images has an optic disk coloboma. Colobomas of the optic nerve head in Collies with Collie eye anomaly are caused by faulty closure or fusion (or both) of the embryonic ventral (i.e. fetal) fissure of the optic stalk and cup; peripapillary colobomas originate from orbital cysts. Optic disk colobomas in Collies may be small and hard to differentiate from a deep, physiologic cup (48c), or they may be very large in diameter (48a). They may be 'typical' at the six o'clock position or 'atypical' at the nasal or temporal disk margin. (48b). Colobomas are also found in Australian Shepherd Dogs, Shelties, Basenjis, American and English Cocker Spaniels, Norfolk Terriers, Huskies, Tibetan Spaniels, Irish Setters, Labrador and Golden Retrievers, Whippets, Samoyeds, Malamutes, Beagles, Bernese Mountain Dogs, Flat-Coated Retrievers, and German Shepherd Dogs.

49 The cornea of a two-year-old German Shepherd Dog (GSD) is shown (49a). The lesion started from the lateral aspect of the cornea and progressed to cover the whole cornea.

i. Describe the lesions.

ii. What is your diagnosis, and what is the etiology of this keratopathy?

iii. What is the treatment?

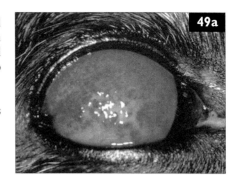

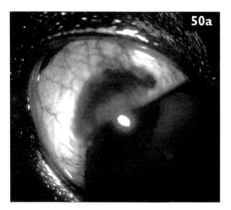

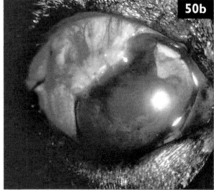

50 An eight-year-old Dachshund is presented with a pigmented mass in the sclera near the limbus (50a). Some corneal invasion is occurring. The conjunctiva is movable over the scleral portion of the lesion.

i. What is the most likely diagnosis?

ii. What is present one-day postoperatively (50b)?

iii. What do the histologic results display (50c)?

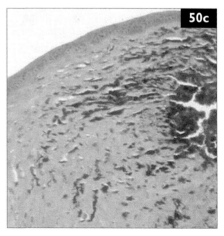

49 i. There are multiple raised, red masses and vascularization covering the whole cornea.

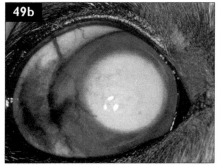

ii. Chronic superficial keratitis (CSK) (pannus). CSK is a progressive, bilateral, inflammatory, and potentially blinding disease of the canine cornea. Clinically, pannus is manifested initially at the temporal or inferior temporal limbus. Vascularization and pigmentation progress centrally (as seen in **49a**) without therapy until the entire cornea becomes vascularized, pigmented, and scarred. GSDs and Greyhounds are most commonly affected with CSK, but it can occur in any breed. Both the incidence and severity of pannus increase at higher altitudes (>1500 meters). In GSDs affected at a fairly young age (1–5 years), the condition is usually rapidly progressive and severe. In those GSDs first affected later in life (4–6 years), however, the lesions appear be less severe and progressive. Greyhounds tend to be affected at less than 2–3 years, and exhibit milder lesions. The cause of CSK in the dog may be an immune-mediated disease against viral or corneal antigens. CSK must be distinguished from pigmentary keratitis due to other causes (e.g. KCS).

iii. Pannus can usually be controlled, but it cannot be cured. Initial therapy consists of topical corticosteroids (0.1% dexamethasone or 1.0% prednisolone 3–4 times daily for 3–4 weeks), followed by a reduced medical maintenance schedule (**49b**). Topical cyclosporin A (0.2–1.0%) can also be an effective treatment.

50 i. A melanoma, which can arise from melanocytes in the limbus or can present from intraocular melanomas invading through the sclera.

ii. A blood clot from hyphema. The limbal melanoma was surgically excised and covered with a conjunctival flap. Six weeks postoperatively the hyphema has resolved and the surgical site is quiet.

iii. Pigmented cells are found invading the cornea (to the left) at the level of the midstroma. The majority of the tumor is in the sclera (on the right).

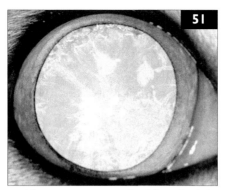

51 This adult six-year-old cat was presented with an incipient cataract (51).
i. What are the possible etiologies for this cataract?
ii. What are the changes associated with an incipient cataract?
iii. What clinical signs may be associated with cataracts?
iv. What are the treatment options for this cat?

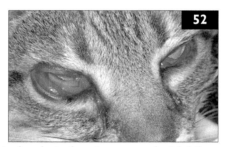

52 An adult domestic shorthaired cat is presented with bilateral, severe swelling of the conjunctiva (52). The right eye is more severely affected than the left, but they are equally painful. Ophthalmic examination reveals no corneal abnormalities. The owner claims that the cat has had redness to its eyes in the past, but never swelling of this magnitude.
i. What are the common causes of feline conjunctivitis?
ii. How will you determine the cause of this cat's conjunctivitis?
iii. How will you treat this cat?

51 i. Cataracts in the cat are usually secondary to trauma, anterior uveitis, glaucoma, metabolic diseases, or lens luxation. Traumatic cataracts are usually focal and slowly progressive. Diabetic metabolic cataracts in cats are less frequent than in diabetic dogs. Other metabolic cataracts in cats can be associated with hypocalcemia from hypoparathyroidism. Cataracts associated with lens luxations are noted as diffuse subcapsular cortical opacities. Uveitis-induced cataracts are also common in cats.

ii. An incipient cataract is an early cataractous change and is usually associated with the cortical, subcortical, and Y suture lines (see case **224**).

iii. Sudden cataract formation is associated with blindness. Cataracts from anterior uveitis may be associated with clinical signs such as aqueous flare, anterior synechiae, rubeosis irides, and iris bombé (see case **215**).

iv. Uveitis can be treated with topical steroids. If the cataract progresses to maturation, it can be removed surgically.

52 i. Conjunctivitis can be frequently caused by feline herpesvirus-1. The virus affects epithelial cells of the respiratory tract, conjunctiva, and cornea. The disease initially affects the youngest of populations, causing sneezing, coughing, and nasal discharge along with fever and generalized malaise. Once infected, the virus can become latent and recur in times of stress. Herpesvirus conjunctivitis can be severe and result in conjunctival ulcerations. *Chlamydophila felis* is an intracellular bacterium that is also a common cause of conjunctivitis in cats. Acute infection leads to conjunctivitis, with possible nasal discharge and sneezing. The conjunctivitis is initially unilateral, but often progresses to bilateral. Calicivirus is an RNA virus that is common in kittens. The virus is specific to the respiratory tract, but can cause conjunctivitis. In most cats the virus is self-limiting.

ii. Cytology and response to therapy.

iii. Herpesviral infections are best treated with antiviral drugs and lysine supplementation. Lysine acts as a competitive inhibitor to arginine, which is an essential amino acid for the herpesvirus. Once infection is apparent, recurrences are likely. Recurrences can include conjunctivitis or the cat may present with characteristic corneal plaques. Chlamydial and mycoplasmal infections are treated with topical and/or oral tetracycline. Vaccination is the best method of prevention for herpesvirus. Calicivirus is fortunately self-limiting because no specific antiviral treatment yet exists for this RNA virus.

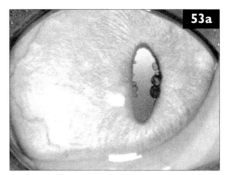

53 A two-year-old neutered Siamese cat was presented for annual examination. Multiple spherical structures were observed at the pupil margins and tapetal reflection could be observed through the tiny spherical structures (53a).
i. What is the diagnosis and significance of these dark structures?
ii. Does this require treatment?

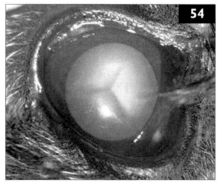

54 A 10-year-old Toy Poodle is presented with progressive blindness. A mydriatic has been applied (54).
i. Describe the lesion.
ii. What is the diagnosis?
iii. What is the treatment?
iv. What is the prognosis for return of vision?

53 i. The spherical structures are uveal cysts. They may arise from the posterior pigment epithelium of the iris or from the inner ciliary body epithelium, and can be congenital or acquired (53b, histologic view ×100). They are remnants of the embryonic optic vesicle and contain a viscous fluid. Uveal cysts are identified by their spherical shape and translucency when illuminated with an intense, focal light source, and are fre-

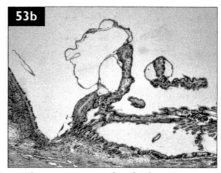

quently positioned at the pupillary margins. These cysts may be thick walled and therefore may not readily transilluminate. Tumors are solid, while cysts are hollow. Iridal cysts may be confused with early melanomas.

ii. Treatment is not usually necessary, but if the cyst is big enough to impair vision, obstruct aqueous flow, or mechanically damage the corneal endothelium, treatment may be indicated. The least invasive method of treatment is the use of a diode laser to achieve rupture and coagulation of the cyst.

54 i. There is a white to blue lens with a separation of the lens fibers and formation of a cleft along the anterior 'Y' suture. There is no tapetal reflection showing.

ii. A mature cataract. The lens fibers are swollen as shown by the Y suture cleft. Compare this cataract with that in case 224, which also involved the suture lines. In that instance the cataract was early in development or incipient.

iii. This cataract is blinding. Most of the lens fibers have become swollen and have begun to break apart in a manner seen in 100b. The treatment to restore vision is phacoemulsification cataract surgery. There is no medical therapy to restore vision lost from cataracts.

iv. Prognosis for return to vision is good with surgery. Prior to surgery, ocular ultrasound and electroretinography are strongly recommended. Ocular ultrasound is used to look for retinal detachments, posterior capsular anomalies (rupture, vascular remnants), and intraocular neoplasia. A fundic examination cannot, however, be performed on a dog with mature cataracts, so electroretinography is used to test retinal function.

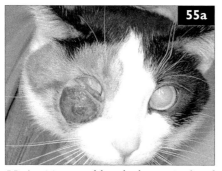
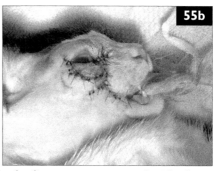

55 An 11-year-old male domestic shorthaired calico cat was presented with a large mass associated with his lower right eyelid (55a). The owner had noticed a raised ulcerative region along the lower eyelid several months previously. As the cat was an outdoor cat, the owner thought the mass was a slow-healing wound that was continually being irritated by the animal.

i. What are the differential diagnoses for the lid lesion in this cat?
ii. What therapy was performed (55b)?

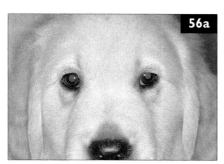
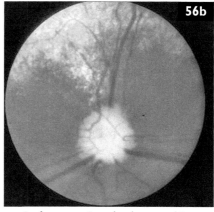

56 A Golden Retriever puppy (56a) has come in for a routine check up and is seen to have a blue tapetal fundus (56b).

i. Is this puppy's fundic examination, as depicted in 56b, normal or abnormal?
ii. This puppy is probably less than what age?
iii. At about what age does the adult tapetal color and structure become fully manifested?

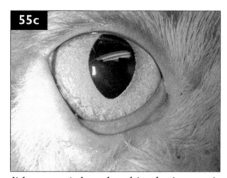

55 i. Diagnosis of eyelid tumors is based on histologic examination. Squamous cell carcinoma (SCC) is the most common eyelid neoplasm in cats. It is thought to be associated with prolonged exposure to actinic radiation and is most prevalent in older white cats. SCC appears clinically as an ulcerative lesion. Basal cell carcinoma can also affect eyelids in the cat. As with SCC, there is a tendency for basal cell carcinoma to become ulcerated. They are usually benign. Mast cell tumors are also found in the eyelids of cats. They can be raised, focal, and are often nonulcerated. Fibrosarcoma of the feline eyelid can be solitary or multicentric, nodular, and often ulcerated. Eyelid fibrosarcomas in younger cats can be caused by feline sarcoma virus (FeSV). The prognosis for life of cats with FeSV-induced tumors is poor, as these cats are feline leukemia virus positive.
ii. A rotating skin flap involving the lip margin was used to remove the SCC in this cat. The result is shown (55c).

56 i. Normal. At around 7–8 weeks of age the blue tapetum is granular in appearance. The optic nerve and retinal vessels all appear normal. The darker spot in the central area of the disc is known as the physiologic cup, and is also normal.
ii. Probably <10 weeks of age.
iii. By about 3–4 months of age.

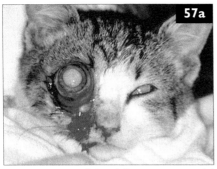
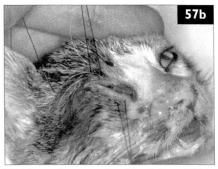

57 Proptosis of the right eye occurred in this kitten due to a dog bite injury (57a). Direct and indirect pupillary light reflexes (PLRs) in this eye are absent.
i. What is the prognosis for vision of the proptosed globe in this cat, and why?
ii. What other clinical signs are associated with a proptosed globe?
iii. What possible long-term sequelae might result from a proptosed globe?
iv. Describe the surgical procedure carried out to replace the globe (57b).

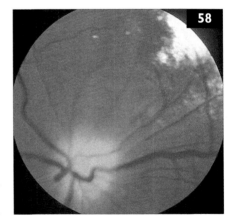

58 A swollen optic nerve is found in a blind dog (58). This adult Border Collie presented for blindness of both eyes and was diagnosed with optic neuritis secondary to granulomatous meningo-encephalitis (GME).
i. What is the presumptive etiology for GME?
ii. What ocular clinical signs are associated with this disease?
iii. What would evaluation of a cerebrospinal fluid (CSF) tap of a dog with GME reveal?
iv. What are the three described classical forms of GME?
v. What diagnostic procedures are best suited for diagnosing GME?
vi. What is the treatment of choice for GME?
vii. What is the prognosis for vision, as well as the prognosis for survival, in a dog with GME?

57 i. Poor, as indicated by the failed PLRs in the globe.

ii. Severe head trauma, fractures of the skull and orbit, corneal perforation/ulceration, and hyphema.

iii. Blindness, keratoconjunctivitis sicca, exposure keratitis, lagophthalmos, exotropia, decreased corneal sensitivity, strabismus, glaucoma, and phthisis bulbi.

iv. The cat is placed under general anesthesia and an artificial tear lubricant used to lubricate the globe. Horizontal mattress sutures are placed through the eyelid margins, and the upper and lower lids are pulled rostrally, dorsally, and ventrally to get them in front of the globe (57b). A temporary tarsorrhaphy is then placed using 4-0 monofilament nonabsorbable suture material and horizontal mattress sutures and stents. The medial canthal area should be exempted from being incorporated into the tarsorrhaphy so that the owner can administer medications. The temporary tarsorrhaphy should be left in place for at least one week.

58 i. It is an idiopathic (possible immune-mediated), nonsuppurative inflammatory disease. GME may be an unusual form of lymphoma.

ii. Ocular signs include acute blindness, peripapillary edema, optic neuritis, dilated pupils, retinal detachment, petechial hemorrhages, uveitis, and secondary glaucoma (see case 206).

iii. CSF fluid may be normal if there is no disruption of the blood–brain barrier, but the classic presentation is a mononuclear pleocytosis with elevated protein.

iv. The focal form that mimics a space-occupying mass, which is associated with a slower onset and progression; the multifocal form, which progresses more rapidly than the focal form and has an acute onset and multifocal neurological involvement; and the ocular form, which has marked nonsuppurative inflammatory infiltrates and granuloma formations within the optic nerve and retina.

v. Procedures include a CSF tap with cytology and culture, and CT or MRI. CT scan findings of a patient with GME include contrast-enhanced lesions, hydrocephalus, edema of the optic nerve, asymmetry of the lateral ventricles, and deviation of the falx cerebri.

vi. An immunosuppressive dose of corticosteroids, which is tapered over many months. In some cases chemotherapeutic agents are used in conjunction with corticosteroids.

vii. There is a very poor prognosis for vision, as well as for long-term survival.

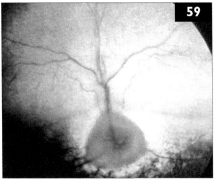

59 This fundus photograph (59) is from an adult Australian Shepherd Dog that was diagnosed with progressive retinal atrophy (PRA).
i. What are the clinical manifestations of PRA?
ii. What is the clinical history that accompanies a dog with PRA?
iii. What other structures in the eye, other than the retina, are affected by PRA?
iv. What is the inheritance of PRA?
v. What diagnostic test can be performed to help with confirmation of PRA?

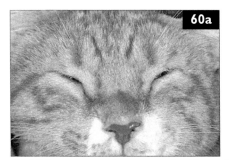
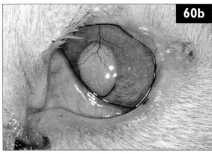

60 This young cat is presented with squinting in both eyes (60a, b).
i. What are the domestic breeds in which this lid condition has been reported?
ii. Is this condition usually unilateral or bilateral?
iii. What are the clinical signs associated with a cat with that has this lid problem? (Use 60b as a guide.)
iv. This lid condition can be associated with what other developmental anomalies?
v. What is the classic surgical technique used to correct this problem?
vi. What are some common complications that can occur and need to be corrected with surgical repair of this condition?

59 i. They include sluggish pupillary light reflexes, retinal atrophy, tapetal hyperreflectivity, and attenuation of retinal blood vessels. Optic nerve head atrophy occurs due to ganglion cell death. Mottling of the nontapetal region is noted in the advanced stage of the disease. PRA is a bilateral disease.

ii. The owners have noted changes in their dog's night vision (nyctalopia) that has become progressively worse with time. Eventually, they also notice a loss of day vision. These changes may occur over several months to years until the dog is blind.

iii. The vitreous degenerates and liquefies in some dogs with PRA. Cataracts are also a common occurrence with PRA due to anterior migration of retinal toxins from the degenerating retina to the posterior lens.

iv. The inheritance varies from autosomal recessive to dominant, and is breed dependent. Genetic testing is available for many dog breeds.

v. Electroretinography can be performed to evaluate retinal function. Early changes show decreases in the b-wave amplitude, while the implicit times are normal. The rods are affected first in PRA, and then the cones.

60 i. This cat has eyelid agenesis, which has been reported in domestic shorthaired cats, Persians, and Burmese.

ii. Usually bilateral.

iii. The area of agenesis (or coloboma) is an area of abnormal eyelid margin development usually noted in the lateral portion of the upper lid, as in **60b**. The patient can develop exposure keratitis, corneal ulceration from exposure, trichiasis, a vascular response secondary to exposure or ulceration, dry eye, and secondary infections.

iv. Colobomas of the choroid and optic nerve. Persistent pupillary membranes and retinal dysplasia may also be present.

v. The Roberts and Bistner procedure is the classic surgical technique where a flap of skin, the orbicularis oculi muscle, and the tarsus are rotated from the inferior eyelid to the superior eyelid to replace the defect. A modification of this technique by Dziezyc and Millichamp was created where a nictitating membrane pedicle is also rotated to the defect to provide conjunctiva to the inner portion of the newly created lid margin.

vi. Upper eyelid hairs may touch the cornea with the rotating flap.

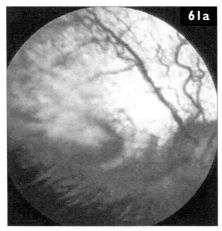

61 The fundus view of the left eye of a young Collie that has Collie eye anomaly (CEA) is shown (**61a**). What is CEA?

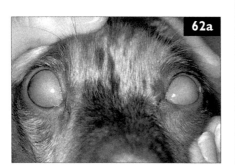

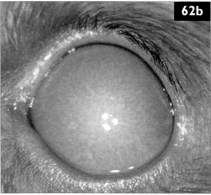

62 A three-year-old female Dachshund presents with a 12-hour history of blue, painful eyes and poor vision. On examination there is moderate to severe corneal edema and anisocoria (**62a, b**).
i. What are the differentials for acute corneal edema?
ii. What additional diagnostics may be helpful?
iii. What are the treatment options?

61 CEA is inherited as a simple auto-somal recessive condition and its expression varies between dogs. The condition is bilateral, although there may be an asymmetry to the lesions present. The disease is generally non-progressive, although eyes with colobomas can infrequently progress to retinal detachment. Reports indicate approximately 85% of Collies (Rough/Smooth) are clinically affected, but this number is declining. Approximately 5–10% of Shetland Sheepdogs have CEA.

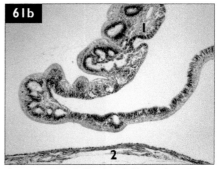

Ophthalmic examination can reveal microphthalmia, focal choroidal hypoplasia located slightly superior and temporal to the optic disk (61a), optic disk coloboma, scleral ectasia, and retinal detachment. The retina has detached from the choroid in this young dog (61b, 1 = retina; 2 = choroid). The choroidal hypoplasia looks like a 'pale' area of varying size dorsal and lateral to the optic disk. It is an area of retinal pigmented epithelium and choroidal hypopigmentation, tapetal hypoplasia, and choroidal dysplasia. Choroidal hypoplasia is found in all eyes with CEA. The retina is atrophic over the area of hypoplasia. Colobomas are severe pits or holes involving the layers of the retina, choroid, sclera, and optic nerve. They may be seen in 30% of dogs with CEA. Large colobomas of the optic disk are associated with visual deficits and may progress to retinal detachment. Retinal detachments are present in 5–10% of the cases. Retinal or vitreous hemorrhage is noticed in 3–4% of CEA eyes.

62 i. Differentials include corneal ulcers, glaucoma, anterior uveitis, and anterior lens luxation (see cases 34 and 116).
ii. Moderate to severe corneal edema makes examination of the inside of the eye difficult. A slit beam was essential in finding the edge of the anteriorly luxated lenses in this dog. Ocular ultrasound can help in determining lens location.
iii. Treatment options for anterior lens luxation are both medical and surgical. An intracapsular lens extraction is generally the recommended surgery to remove the lens if corneal edema is present.

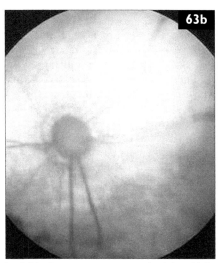

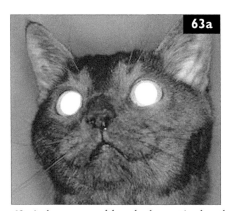

63 A three-year-old male domestic shorthaired black cat was presented with widely dilated pupils (63a). The owner felt that he seemed to have lost his vision. She had noticed these changes in the past day and wondered whether it had any relationship to his recent treatment for urinary tract obstruction. He did not respond to a menace test and had slow and incomplete pupillary light reflexes. Ophthalmoscopic examination revealed tapetal hyperreflectivity and considerable attenuation of the retinal blood vessels (63b). Scattered rust-colored spots were also apparent within the tapetal fundus. What are the differential diagnoses for the retinal degeneration in this cat?

64 This dog was referred to a veterinary ophthalmologist after three weeks of medical therapy for a superficial ulcer with no progress in healing (64). On presentation, an axial superficial ulcer (about 30% of corneal surface in size) was observed.

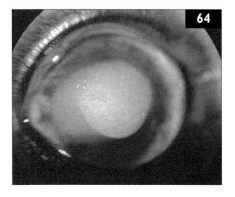

i. Describe the pathophysiology of spontaneous chronic corneal epithelial defects (SCCEDs) (also known as indolent ulcers or 'Boxer ulcers').
ii. How would you diagnose a SCCED?

63 Inherited, idiopathic, toxic, or associated with taurine deficiency. A rod-cone dysplasia and a rod-cone degeneration have been described in the Abyssinian breed, with the former occurring as early as one month after birth, and the latter beginning at 1.5–2.0 years of age and taking another 2–4 years to progress to complete blindness. Taurine is an essential dietary requirement in cats, as they are unable to synthesize taurine from its precursor cysteine. Taurine is a cell membrane stabilizer and neurotransmitter and is highly concentrated within the photoreceptors. Taurine depletion thus leads to retinal degeneration.

This cat had been treated for urinary obstruction with enrofloxacin, which has recently been associated with a rare adverse ophthalmic toxicity causing an acute, irreversible retinal degeneration in cats. The reported incidence of this adverse reaction is 1 in 122,414 treated cats (i.e. 0.0008%). Adherence to the manufacturer's current recommendation for enrofloxacin dosage in cats of 2.5 mg/kg BID orally is advisable, but may still be too high for some aged cats. There is a remote possibility that vision can return if enrofloxacin is stopped as soon as mydriasis and blindness are observed. Marbofloxacin has been shown not to be as toxic and is safer to use in cats.

64 i. SCCEDs are chronic superficial epithelial ulcers that fail to resolve through normal wound healing processes. They have been documented in almost every canine breed. It is likely that the initiating event in dogs is minor superficial trauma. Histology shows the epithelium to be poorly attached to the underlying corneal stroma and there is evidence of dysmaturation or loss of the normal epithelial architecture. A variable amount of stromal fibroplasia, vascularization, and leukocytic infiltrate occurs. There is either no epithelial basement membrane or only small discontinuous segments of basement membrane on the surface of the exposed stroma. A hyalinized acellular zone composed of collagen fibrils admixed with an ill-defied amorphous or fine fibrillar material and fibrin is present on the SCCED surface.
ii. A SCCED should be considered in any middle-aged and older dog with a superficial nonhealing ulcer. Underlying causes for a nonhealing ulcer include lid abnormalities such as lid tumors, ectopic cilia, entropion and lagophthalmia, foreign bodies, infection, tear film abnormalities, exposure from poor lid conformation, paralysis of lids, neurotrophic keratitis, exophthalmia or buphthalmia, or corneal edema leading to bullous keratopathy. If no underlying causes of nonhealing are found in a superficial ulcer with loose or redundant epithelial edges, such that fluorescein stain pools underneath a seemingly intact epithelium, then a diagnosis of SCCED can be made.

65 How would you treat the dog in 64?

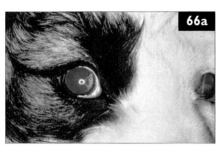

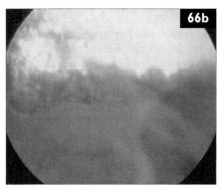

66 This male Border Collie is brought to the clinic with a fixed and dilated pupil in both eyes (66a). The fundic image of the right eye is shown (66b).
i. What is the diagnosis and pathogenesis?
ii. What would the clinical findings be on retinal examination?
iii. What specific breeds may be at risk for the condition that is present in this animal?

67 This is a fundus photograph (67) of a three-year-old domestic shorthaired cat that presented with chorioretinitis.
i. Are these lesions active or inactive?
ii. What are the etiologies for chorioretinitis in the cat?

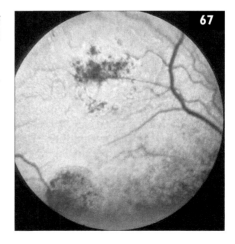

65 Débridement of loose epithelium with a dry, sterile cotton-tipped swab after application of topical anesthesia can be repeated at 21-day intervals. Punctate (65a) or grid keratotomy (65b) using a 20G needle to aid adhesion can be performed after epithelial débridement. Superficial keratectomy is more invasive and requires general anesthesia and may cause more scarring, but is successful in a majority of the cases. Application of a soft contact lens after any of these procedures will reduce frictional irritation from the eyelids, improve comfort, and help with healing. Topical corticosteroids should be avoided, as they can decrease the rate of corneal wound healing and decrease host defense mechanisms. Medical therapy includes topical broad-spectrum antibiotics, serum, and hypertonics such as 5% NaCl.

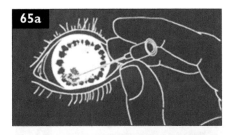

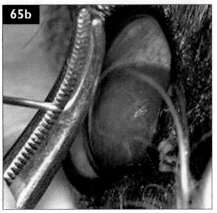

66 i. Optic nerve aplasia. This condition is caused by the complete absence of retinal ganglion cells and the ganglion axons that would normally form the optic nerve.
ii. Retinal examination would reveal an absence of the optic nerve as well as retinal vessels. Anatomically, the optic nerve is entirely absent. Only a small cluster of supportive tissue might be observed when examining this region histologically.
iii. Irish Wolfhound and Beagle.

67 i. The lesions look inactive based on the sharp and distinct borders of the lesions. There is atrophy of the tapetal neural retina in this cat, which is noted by hyperreflectivity. The retinal pigmented epithelium was affected by the disease such that the center of the lesion is pigmented. Active chorioretinal lesions have indistinct borders due to retinal edema (see case 186).
ii. Blastomycosis, histoplasmosis, cryptococcosis, feline infectious peritonitis, and mycobacteriosis are associated with granulomatous chorioretinitis in cats.

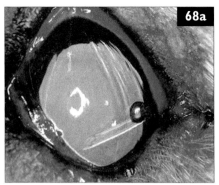
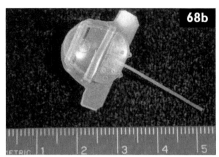

68 This dog has had surgery for glaucoma.
i. What is the name and function of the device seen in the anterior chamber of this dog's eye (**68a**) and illustrated in **68b**?
ii. What is the indication for this type of surgical procedure?
iii. What is the lowest intraocular pressure that this device is designed to permit?
iv. What is a common complication after placement of gonioimplants in dogs?

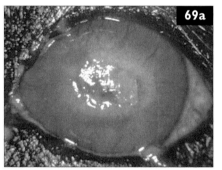
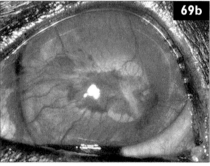

69 A dog presents with keratoconjunctivitis siccca and reduced corneal sensation (**69a**). The same eye is shown as it appeared two months later (**69b**).
i. Describe the clinical findings based on the original presentation (**69a**).
ii. What is the sensory innervation of the cornea?
iii. What problems arise when there is dysfunction of the corneal sensory nerves?
iv. What examination techniques can be used to evaluate corneal sensitivity?
v. What can cause damage to the sensory innervation of the cornea?
vi. What are some general treatment options that should be implemented in a dog with this condition?

68 i. An Ahmed valve, which is designed to bypass the blocked iridocorneal angle and shunt aqueous humor into the subconjunctival space. The cornea is wrinkled due to low intraocular pressure (IOP) (**68a**).
ii. This type of valve is surgically implanted in eyes with glaucoma that have an IOP that is not responsive to medical therapy.
iii. Unidirectional valved systems are designed to permit passage of aqueous humor at approximately 10–12 mmHg.
iv. The tubing can become blocked with fibrin and therefore unable to shunt aqueous humor out of the anterior chamber.

69 i. There is a pink to red area of granulation tissue associated with the axial cornea. Vascularization is present over 360 degrees. The cornea is edematous peripheral to the central lesion. The peripheral cornea is clear enough to see the iris and pupil.
ii. The long ciliary nerves, which are derived from the ophthalmic division of the trigeminal nerve (cranial nerve V).
iii. A decreased blink response and an increased evaporation of the precorneal tear film. Corneal healing is also slowed.
iv. The frequency of the blink reflex should be assessed, as a reduction in blinking may indicate reduced corneal sensitivity. Corneal sensitivity can be evaluated by touching the cornea with a small piece of cotton. If the sensitivity is normal, the patient will blink and retract the globe, causing protrusion of the third eyelid. A Cochet–Bonnet esthesiometer can also be used to assess corneal sensitivity. An adjustable nylon filament is used to stimulate the cornea. When a blink reflex is only elicited with a short filament, corneal sensation is reduced. When a long filament elicits a blink reflex, corneal sensation is normal.
v. Trauma to the head. This condition is also commonly present in brachycephalic dogs and diabetic animals.
vi. Artificial tears and serum are used to protect the insensitive cornea. A third eyelid flap or temporary tarsorrhaphy may also provide some protection of the cornea when decreased corneal sensitivity is present.

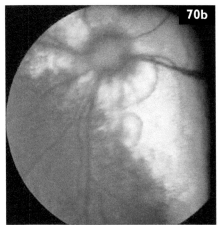

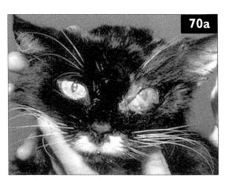

70 A 15-year-old cat presents with a two-week history of exophthalmos and nictitans protrusion (70a) as well as the funduscopic changes shown (70b).
i. What are the differentials for feline exophthalmos?
ii. Describe the fundic lesions.
iii. What is the prognosis for feline orbital tumors?

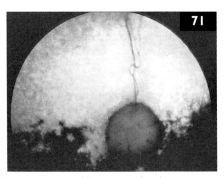

71 This adult Poodle was presented because of a decrease in vision at night, but it still had some vision during the day.
i. What clinical signs are noted in 71?
ii. What is the most likely inherited disease that is being depicted in this Poodle?
iii. What are the clinical complaints from an owner with a dog that suffers from this disease?
iv. What diagnostic test should be performed to confirm the diagnosis?

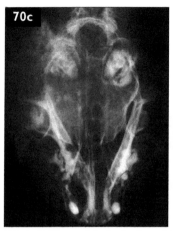
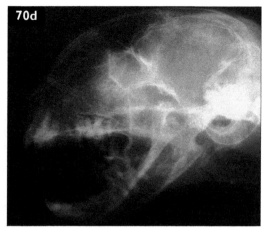

70 i. Differentials include orbital abscess, orbital cellulitis, orbital emphysema, orbital tumor, extraorbital tumor (sinus or nasal), and trauma.

ii. There are two focal areas of retinal detachment in the tapetum ventral to the optic nerve head. Retinal detachment may occur in this cat due to the mechanical pressure from an orbital mass, the mass irritating the globe, or vascular compromise to the globe.

iii. Poor. Approximately 90% of orbital tumors are malignant. A complete work-up for metastasis is recommended prior to surgery. Radiography (70c, d) reveals significant amounts of bony erosion in the orbital region of this cat with orbital osteosarcoma.

71 i. There is retinal vessel attenuation and a focal area of hyperreflectivity noted dorsal, temporal, and nasal to the optic nerve. The optic nerve appears slightly small and dark.

ii. Progressive retinal atrophy (PRA).

iii. Decreased vision at night or in dim light (nyctalopia) in both eyes is noted in dogs with PRA. The pupillary light reflex is sluggish and there is a larger resting pupil than normal. Dogs with PRA may develop secondary cataracts in the advanced stages of this disease.

iv. Electroretinography can be performed to evaluate for PRA, as well as genetic blood testing to identify affected dogs (see case **59**).

72 A five-year-old domestic shorthaired cat was presented for ocular examination after a fight with another cat (72a).
i. Describe the findings and differential diagnosis.
ii. How would you treat this condition?

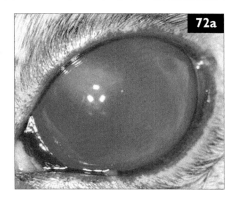

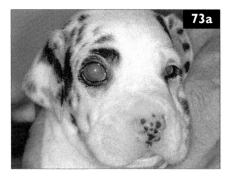

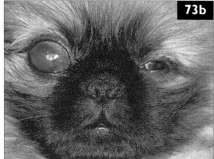

73 From time to time, young pets brought to the clinic can have significant differences with regard to the size of their right and left eye. The difference in the size of an animal's eyes is usually the result of one being abnormally larger than the other. There also may be times when one or both eyes can be observably smaller than normal. Three examples (two puppies and one kitten) are shown (73a–c) where one eye is substantially larger than the other. What condition is present in these animals?

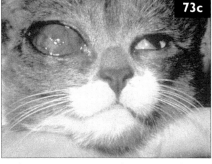

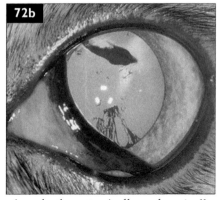

72 i. There is a corneal lesion with severe local corneal edema. There is hyphema in the anterior chamber and the iris and the pupil cannot be identified. Hyphema can be caused by trauma, retinal detachment, neoplasia, uveitis (due to systemic diseases or other reasons), coagulopathies, vasculitis (immune-mediated or secondary to rickettsial diseases), systemic hypertension, or parasite migration, and can be secondary to congenital ocular defects (such as in Collie eye anomaly).

ii. Broad-spectrum antibiotics should be given both systemically and topically. Uveitis should be treated aggressively with systemic and topical anti-inflammatory drugs. Atropine should be given topically to prevent synechiae and discomfort. Tissue plasminogen activator may be necessary to digest fibrin in the anterior chamber. Corneal lacerations with leakage of aqueous humor require corneal suturing and the possible placement of a conjunctival graft to seal the corneal fistula and promote healing. Damage to the lens may lead to lens-induced uveitis and cataract formation. In this case the hyphema cleared almost completely 13 days after initiation of medical therapy, and the iris and pupil could be clearly seen (72b). A small blood clot and fibrin with adjacent focal cataractous changes are present on the dorsal aspect of the anterior lens capsule, Cataracts may form in some eyes following lens capsule rupture and require surgical removal by an ophthalmologist.

73 Buphthalmos, which is generally found with advanced chronic glaucoma. In kittens and puppies, congenital glaucoma is usually secondary to malformation of the iridocorneal angle and/or dysgenesis of the structures of the anterior segment. The eyes of young animals tend to enlarge more rapidly and more severely when glaucoma is present. There is no treatment other than enucleation if the lids cannot protect the cornea.

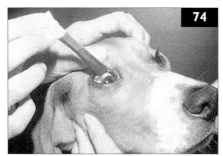

74 The application of fluorescein dye (**74**) may be performed during an ophthalmic examination (e.g. cases **21, 153, 156**) to determine the integrity of the corneal epithelium.
i. Which layer(s) of the cornea does fluorescein stain?
ii. What other ophthalmic uses are there for fluorescein dye?

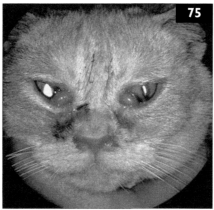

75 The owner of this male cat (**75**) says she does not know what is wrong, but when her cat came home after being away for a couple of days, his eyes were all red and swollen. She thinks he might have been in a fight.
i. What do you tell the owner is wrong with her cat?
ii. What causes this condition in cats?
iii. What do you recommend as treatment?

74 i. The cornea has four layers: the epithelium, stroma, Descemet's membrane, and the endothelium. The corneal epithelium is hydrophobic/lipophilic and prevents any appreciable penetration of fluorescein. The water-soluble fluorescein dye will stain the corneal stroma, but will not stain a healthy intact epithelium or Descemet's membrane. In the presence of a corneal epithelial defect or ulcer, the dye rapidly diffuses into the corneal stroma.

ii. The passage of fluorescein from the eye to the external nares evaluates the patency of the nasolacrimal system (Jones I test). A strip of fluorescein is moistened with a few drops of sterile eyewash and touched to the upper bulbar conjunctiva. The dye usually appears at the external nares within five minutes in dogs and cats. Fluorescein may exit more readily into the nasopharynx in cats and brachycephalic dogs. The animal's tongue and saliva should also be examined in these cases. Fluorescein can also be used to look for corneal fistulas, leaking sutures, and leaking descemetoceles with the Seidel's test. Fluorescein is applied to the cornea and examined for a change in color associated with aqueous humor dilution of the fluorescein. The tear film breakup time can also be evaluated with fluorescein stain. After application of fluorescein to the cornea, the eyelids are held open to prevent blinking, and the cornea observed for the appearance of dark areas in the fluorescein stain. It should take >15–20 seconds for these dark areas to appear if the tear film integrity is stable, and be very quick if there is a tear film problem.

75 i. This cat has bilateral eversion or prolapse of the gland of the nictitans, a condition commonly referred to as 'cherry eye'.

ii. This condition in cats occurs especially in the Burmese breed. The eversion of the nictitans and prolapse of the gland is caused by folding of the narrow stem of cartilage near the gland. The cause of the cartilage folding is unknown. It has been suggested that there is deterioration of the attachments between the cartilage and the deep orbital fascia. This condition is not only unsightly to the owner, but can be uncomfortable and possibly cause corneal ulceration in the patient.

iii. Eversions of the nictitans gland can be treated by surgical removal or amputation of the hypertrophied gland; however, this is generally no longer recommended due to the risk of decreased tear production and keratoconjunctivitis sicca post gland amputation surgery. Several techniques for surgical replacement of the everted nictitans gland have been described.

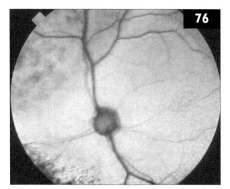

76 A cat is presented with sneezing, difficulty breathing, disorientation, and staggering. Fundic examination reveals chorioretinitis with multiple, slightly raised, gray-yellow exudative lesions (76).
i. What is your diagnosis?
ii. Describe the disease and the ocular manifestations.
iii. What is your treatment recommendation?

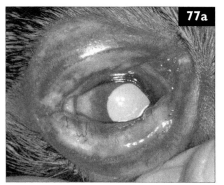
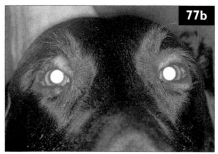

77 A young adult Labrador Retriever is presented with moderate to severe, generalized blepharitis (77a, b). The owner explains that the dog can often be found rubbing his eyes on the carpets. Occasionally, he has moderate epiphora. He is otherwise healthy and on no medications at this time.
i. Explain the possible causes of blepharitis.
ii. How might you determine the cause in this case?
iii. How would you treat this condition for each cause?

76 i. The most likely diagnosis based on the fundic examination is granulomatous chorioretinitis caused by the fungus *Cryptococcus neoformans* (see **186b**).
ii. The fungus is likely contracted by inhalation of infective spores, which can deposit in the upper or lower respiratory tract. Once established in the airways, the infection can spread hematogenously or by tissue invasion. Infections with *C. neoformans* may result from immunosuppression in cats with feline immuno-deficiency virus and feline leukemia virus infection, in dogs with ehrlichiosis, and from chronic glucocorticoid therapy. Eye infections can arise hematogenously or via extension from the brain by the optic nerve. Clinical presentation can range from dilated, unresponsive pupils and blindness to chorioretinitis, anterior uveitis, and retinal damage
iii. While the prognosis for survival with the ocular form of cryptococcosis is fair to good using triazole antifungal drugs, the prognosis for return of vision is guarded to poor due to retinal damage.

77 i. Bacterial, fungal, and parasitic infections, or immune mediated. Bacterial blepharitis is most commonly caused by *Staphylococcus* or *Streptococcus* spp. Mycotic blepharitis results from concurrent skin infection with *Trichophyton* or *Microsporum* spp. Parasitic blepharitis can occur from generalized infection with *Demodex canis* or *Sarcoptes scabiei*. Immune-mediated blepharitis can be seen with pemphigus, uveodermatologic syndrome, and other immune-mediated diseases.
ii. A careful skin scraping of the eyelid, with direct cytology (for *Demodex* or *Sarcoptes* identification) and culture on Sabouraud-dextrose agar (for *Trichophyton* and *Microsporum*). In the presence of lid abscesses and exudates, swabs should be submitted for cytology, culture, and sensitivity.
iii. Bacterial blepharitis is treated with systemic and topical ophthalmic antibiotics consistent with the sensitivity results received. Mycotic blepharitis is treated with thorough cleansing of the area with povidone–iodine scrub in addition to a topical miconazole cream. Systemic antifungals (e.g. ketoconazole) can be useful for stubborn, chronic mycotic blepharitis infections. Demodectic blepharitis is typically self-limited in young dogs, but healing can be aided by treatment with amitraz dips or systemic ivermectin or milbemycin. Sarcoptic blepharitis is best treated with multiple lime sulfur dips and/or amitraz. Ivermectin and selemectin (two doses at 30-day intervals) are also effective. Immune-mediated blepharitis is treated with long-term systemic and topical corticosteroids. Stronger immunosuppressive drugs, such as cyclophosphamide, have also been used in chronic cases.

78 A Maine Coon kitten is examined at the clinic (78).
i. Describe the clinical signs illustrated.
ii. What congenital disease does this Maine Coon kitten have?
iii. Why did this congenital disease develop?

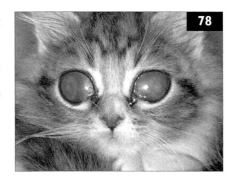

79 A two-year-old male Golden Retriever presents for yearly vaccination. On ophthalmic examination there is a round, brown cystic structure (arrow) free floating in the anterior chamber (79).
i. What is the diagnosis, and where do these structures arise?
ii. What is its significance?

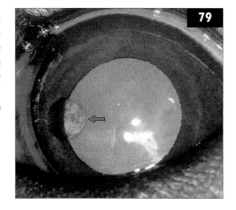

80 Ophthalmic examinations often include the technique being used here (80).
i. What diagnostic technique is being demonstrated in this image?
ii. What are the limitations of this technique?

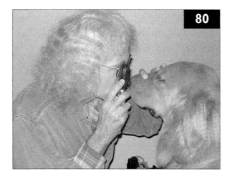

78 i. There is buphthalmia, corneal edema, and keratitis.
ii. Bilateral primary glaucoma.
iii. This bilateral congenital disease developed because of a developmental abnormality of the aqueous humor outflow pathways alone or as part of anterior segment dysgenesis.

79 i. A uveal cyst, which is often seen in the Golden Retriever (compare with case **19**), Labrador Retriever, and Boston Terrier. Uveal cysts arise from either posterior pigmented epithelium of the iris or from the inner ciliary body epithelium (see case **53**).
ii. Uveal cysts are round and usually considered benign. The potential complications to benign cysts are glaucoma (obstruction of outflow) and cyst rupture (pigment then attaching to the corneal endothelium or anterior lens capsule). Careful examination for signs of uveitis in Golden Retrievers with uveal cysts is indicated, since both may occur at the same time in this breed. Note that in this case the cyst is less pigmented than in case **19**. This is most likely the result of it having arisen from the nonpigmented epithelial layer of the ciliary process.

80 i. Direct ophthalmoscopy. A condensing lens is not positioned between the ophthalmoscope and the patient's eye so the examiner has a direct optical image of the patient's eye. The fundus image is highly magnified, real, and upright. The direct ophthalmoscope head offers a range of lenses to enable focusing at various depths within the eye. These lenses are calibrated in diopters and are color coded. The diopter setting is usually started at 0 and adjusted to between +3 (green) and -3 (red) to provide the sharpest image possible. Minor alterations in the setting of the ophthalmoscopic lenses are usually needed to focus on the patient's retina and optic nerve. There are also controls for spot size and brightness. There may be a red-free filter, and a cobalt blue filter is used to look for corneal ulcers. The 'red-free' (do not call it 'green') filter is useful for enhancing the appearance of blood vessels and hemorrhages by making blood show up black.
ii. Penetration of cloudy or partially crystallized media is limited by the relatively low intensity of the instrument's bulb. Because of the extreme magnification, there is a small field of view and examination of the peripheral fundus becomes difficult. Stereopsis is absent and depth of focus is limited. The small working distance between examiner and patient may be hazardous if examining aggressive and frightened animals.

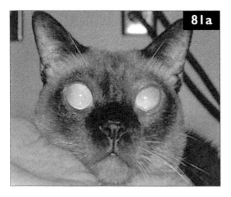

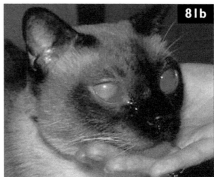

81 A nine-year-old Siamese cat is presented for blindness (81a–c).
i. Describe the lesions.
ii. What is the most likely diagnosis?
iii. Which breeds of cat are predisposed to this condition?
iv. What are the treatment options for these conditions?

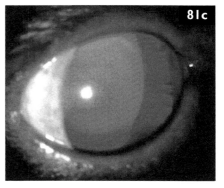

82 A relatively young Doberman Pinscher is presented with these fine opacities in the vitreous humor (82). What is the differential diagnosis for these vitreal opacities?

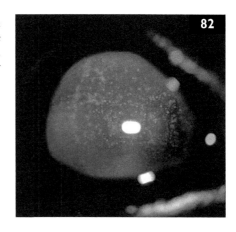

81 i. There is bilateral mydriasis, with green tapetal and red choroidal reflections (see **81a**). When looking at the eyes at an angle, there is a red fundic reflection in the ventral pupil bilaterally (see **81b, c**). In **81c** a lens subluxation is revealed by the presence of a bright red fundic reflection (central), an aphakic crescent, and taut ciliary body processes (right).

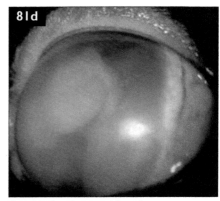

ii. The most likely diagnosis for a Siamese cat that presents blind with dilated pupils is primary glaucoma. Systemic hypertension and retinal disease should also be considered.

iii. Siamese, European Shorthair, Burmese, and Persian breeds.

iv. The treatment options for primary glaucoma are medical (see case 34) and surgical. Surgical therapies for glaucoma include gonioshunts, ciliary body ablation (**81d**, lens rupture following accidental intralenticular injection of gentamicin instead of the vitreous during a ciliary body ablation procedure), cryotherapy, or diode laser), enucleation, and evisceration with prosthetic implant. The treatment options for lens subluxations are medical therapy for uveitis and intraocular pressure increases, and monitoring for complete luxation.

82 Vitreous opacities may be caused by inflammatory vitritis, hemorrhage, asteroid hyalosis, and synchysis scintillans. Retinal detachment, luxated lens, foreign bodies, neoplasms, and parasites (*Dirofilaria*) may also cause vitreal opacities. This case represents a vitreal degeneration termed asteroid hyalosis. Asteroid hyalosis is relatively common in dogs and is often called 'floaters'. Complexes of calcium–lipid crystals attached to the framework of the vitreous oscillate slightly when the eye/head moves. Synchysis scintillans is rare in dogs and is associated with retinal degeneration. The cholesterol crystals in the liquefied vitreous of synchysis scintillans display 'snow flake' movement when the globe moves. There is no therapy for asteroid hyalosis or synchysis scintillans.

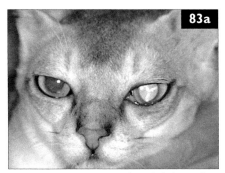

83 A one-year-old Singapura cat is presented with bilateral epiphora of four weeks' duration (83a). The lid margins are normal and there is no conjunctivitis.
i. What diagnostic test should be performed?
ii. If the test is negative, what is the next step?
iii. After these tests, what is the most likely diagnosis?
iv. What are the treatment options?

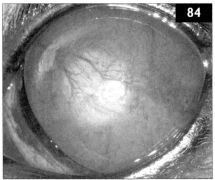

84 A long-haired Dachshund is presented with epiphora and possible vision loss. The owner explains that she has just had the living room remodeled and noticed the dog bumping into the new furniture. Complete ophthalmic examination reveals corneal cloudiness, mild to moderate corneal pigmentation, normal tear production, and corneal neovascularization (84). The cornea is fluorescein negative.
i. What is the diagnosis and etiology?
ii. What are your differential diagnoses?
iii. Describe the pathophysiology of the condition.
iv. How will you treat the eye?

83 i. A Jones test is used to determine patency of the nasolacrimal system. This cat had a negative Jones test.

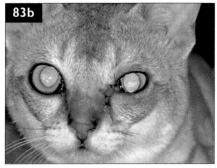

ii. The next step is to cannulate the upper and lower puncta and flush the ducts. There were no duct openings in this cat. There were also no nasal duct openings in either nostril. A dacryocystorhinogram cannot therefore be performed because contrast cannot be injected into the nasolacrimal system.

iii. As there are no openings on the nasal or conjunctival ends of the nasolacrimal system, the most likely diagnosis is nasolacrimal agenesis. Cats that are brachycephalic are most commonly diagnosed with this problem.

iv. The treatment of choice is a conjunctivalrhinostomy (83b) or a conjunctivaloralostomy. A lower puncta is created when an osteotomy is performed into the nasal passage or oral cavity, respectively. The new drainage system is cannulated with silicone tubing and left in place for 4–6 weeks.

84 i. Immune-mediated punctate keratitis, a breed-related corneal disease.

ii. Differentials include pigmentary keratitis, pannus, keratoconjunctivitis sicca, glaucoma, and retinal degeneration.

iii. Immune-mediated punctate keratitis is most common in long-haired Dachshunds, but may occur in any breed of dog. This chronic disease can lead to cloudiness of the entire cornea, pigmentation, and some degree of vision loss. Excessive exposure to ultraviolet radiation may aggravate this condition.

iv. The eye is fluorescein negative and is therefore not ulcerated. However, if ulceration was present, antibiotics would be necessary. In this case, treatment consists of topical cyclosporin A and corticosteroids for extended periods. Therapy may be a lifelong.

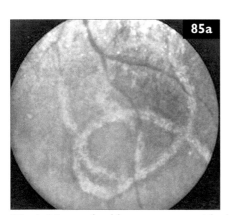

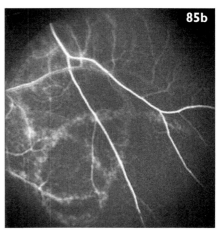

85 A 14-month-old cat presents with the curvilinear tracts seen in these fundic photographs (85a, b).
i. What diagnostic technique has been used to highlight the curvilinear tracts in the retina seen in 85b?
ii. What is the cause of these curvilinear tracts?
iii. Where do these parasites migrate?
iv. What are the most common clinical signs reported by owners of cats with this disease?

86   A six-month-old Shar Pei is presented with epiphora, blepharospasm, and chemosis. Initial examination reveals entropion of the upper and lower eyelids and a protruding descemetocele (86).
i. What steps will you take to examine this puppy and determine the diagnosis?
ii. What are the etiology and pathophysiology of the condition?
iii. Describe the treatment you will recommend.
iv. What follow-up care will be necessary?

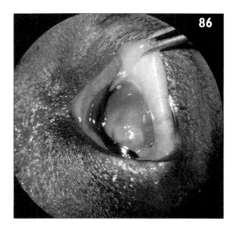

85 i. Fluorescein angiography. Defects in the retinal pigment epithelium from the larval migration allow visualization of the fluorescein dye in the choroid.
ii. Ophthalmomyiasis (see case **95**).

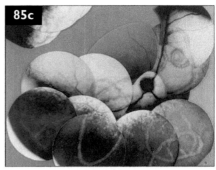

iii. In and around the sensory retina (85c, collage of fundus photographs showing the migratory marks going around the optic nerve).
iv. Usually there are no specific clinical signs and cats are asymptomatic. There have been cases where ophthalmomyiasis has caused anterior uveitis in cats.

86 i. Careful examination of the margins of the eyelids is necessary to look for distichia or ectopic cilia. Fluorescein stain uptake is critical to evaluate corneal ulcers. The stain will not bind to healthy epithelium or to Descemet's membrane. A cobalt blue filtered light enhances the fluorescence and can be helpful in defining the nature of the stain uptake. In this dog, the center of the ulcer did not take up stain, indicating the presence of a descemetocele (see cases **142** and **232**). A culture swab of the ulcer would be warranted to define the most effective antibiotic for this animal.
ii. In breeds with excessive skin folding (e.g. Shar Pei, Bulldog, Chow Chow), moderate to severe entropion with trichiasis often occurs (see case **157**). Irritation by the redundant skin and trichiasis cause blepharospasm and corneal ulceration. Long-term irritation causes scarring and pigmentation of the cornea.
iii. The descemetocele should be treated with a conjunctival graft. The eyelid changes require blepharoplastic procedures. Conjunctival grafts provide physical/structural support, deliver plasma to the injured area, add fibroblasts to the ulcer site, and direct a vascular supply to the corneal lesion.
iv. Conjunctival flaps require trimming approximately 6–8 weeks post surgery to minimize corneal scarring. Trimming of the blood supply requires sedation, topical anesthesia, and tenotomy scissors.

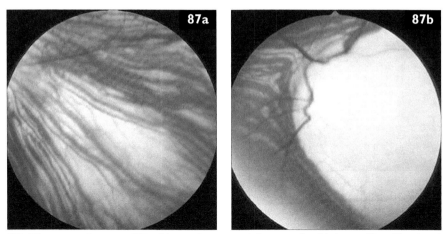

87 These two images (87a, b) are from an eight-month-old Australian Shepherd Dog. Note what is demonstrated in the retina in 87b.
i. Based on these images, what is the diagnosis, and how does it form embryologically?
ii. What is the name of the syndrome associated with these lesions in the Australian Shepherd Dog?
iii. Describe the histologic appearance of these lesions.
iv. What is the inheritance of microphthalmia with this condition in Australian Shepherd Dogs?

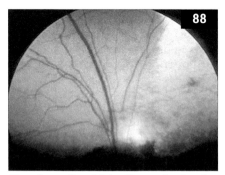

88 This dog has a dilated pupil, which allows the fundus to be seen by direct ophthalmoscopy (88). What is discovered in the direct ophthalmoscopic image?

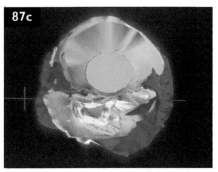

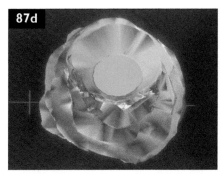

87 i. White equatorial colobomas. Embryologically, colobomas form due to a primary defect in the retinal pigmented epithelium (RPE). This results in focal hypoplasia of the choroid and sclera. This 3-D reconstruction of a young Australian Shepherd Dog eye (87c) shows the absence of some of its RPE (fuchsia color), which led to a subsequent coloboma. The lens is blue, and the outer and inner retinae are green and yellow, respectively. As the loss of choroidal elements mimics the absence of the RPE, the sclera will seal this defect to form a coloboma, but in a less than perfect way (87d).

ii. Merle ocular dysgenesis (MOD), which is accompanied by multiple ocular disorders including micropthalmia, microcornea, heterochromia irides, dyscoria, corectopia, hypoplastic irides, cataracts, retinal detachment, and the colobomas.

iii. They show decreased to absent choroidal vasculature in the location, and a thin and irregular sclera.

iv. MOD in this breed is inherited as an autosomal recessive with incomplete penetrance. Dogs with MOD are homozygous merles with significant white coat color.

88 The retina and optic nerve head (ONH) changes are a result of glaucoma. The ONH is demyelinated, dark, and atrophic. A small region of tapetal hyper-reflectivity is present adjacent to the right side of the optic disk. The optic nerve disc has moved posteriorly in response to elevated intraocular pressure to block the circulation from a short posterior ciliary artery to the retina. As a single short posterior ciliary artery provides blood to specific wedge-shaped regions of retina, the ischemia from such a reduction in the retinal circulation results in retinal edema and an associated wedge-shaped hyporeflective tapetal pattern, as is seen from 9 to 1 o'clock.

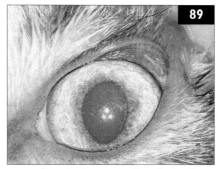

89 A two-year-old neutered male domestic shorthaired cat is presented with an abnormal eyelid margin (89). This cat has been treated on-and-off over the past three months for a lid abscess.
i. What is the most likely diagnosis?
ii. What are the differentials for the eyelid abscess?
iii. What are the treatment options?

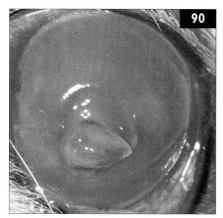

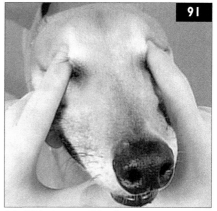

90 A young adult dog (mixed breed) is presented with this condition (90).
i. What is the diagnosis?
ii. What can be done therapeutically?

91 This image (91) shows an examination procedure referred to as retropulsing the globes.
i. Describe the process of globe retropulsion.
ii. What circumstances might arise that would not allow for retropulsion?

89 i. Cicatricial ectropion. The chronic eyelid abscess or pyogranuloma has resolved with a scar (cicatrix). The contraction of the scar has caused the ectropion.
ii. Differentials include neoplasia, meibomian gland adenitis, chalazia (chronic lipid granuloma of meibomian glands), eyelid cysts, eosinophilic keratitis plaques, and eyelid pyogranulomas.
iii. Treatment of the eyelid abscess or pyogranuloma starts with confirmation of the diagnosis. Diagnosis is based on cytologic examination (polymorphonuclear neutrophils, lymphocytes, plasma cells with evidence of chronic inflammation) or excisional biopsy. Treatment is systemic and intralesional injections of antibiotics followed by warm compresses. In this case, after the eyelid pyogranuloma had resolved, a cicatricial ectropion occurred. The treatment of choice for cicatricial ectropion is a simple V to Y blepharoplasty. The procedure requires dissection of the scar tissue, mobilization of the adjacent skin, and suturing of the V into a Y, thus pushing the skin toward the eye.

90 i. This is an iris prolapse with the protruding iris covered in a layer of beige colored fibrin. There may be persistent aqueous humor leakage, which causes a low intraocular presure, shallow anterior chamber, and persistent uveitis, or the corneal perforation may be sealed with iris and fibrin.
ii. If there is a dazzle reflex or a consensual pupillary light reflex to the other eye to indicate a functional retina in this eye, the protruding iris can be amputated and the corneal lesion covered by a corneal transplant or a conjunctival graft. An ocular ultrasound can be beneficial for evaluating retinal function in these cases, but must be carefully performed due to the keratopathy. Infection and uveitis are then treated topically.

91 i. Globe retropulsion is a test used to evaluate orbital volume changes and orbital pain. Gentle digital pressure is applied to the globe with the eyelids closed. The globes should be easily moved posteriorly by this pressure in most dogs, and no signs of pain or discomfort should be observed.
ii. A space-occupying lesion behind the globe, such as an abscess, cellulitis, tumor, or cysts, would prevent the globe from being retropulsed (see cases **9**, **98**, and **166**). Retropulsion of the orbit of small breed dogs and most cats will yield little posterior globe movement, as the orbit is small.

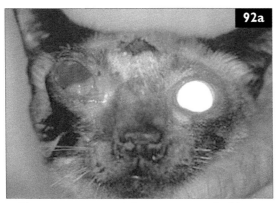

92 A 16-year-old cat presents with a two-month history of progressive exophthalmos and a recent history of hemorrhagic nasal discharge (92a).
i. What part of the physical examination is critical in this cat?
ii. What is the treatment of choice?

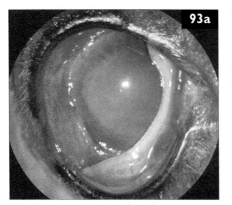 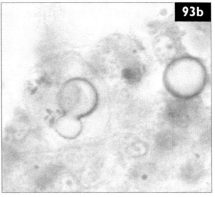

93 You are presented with a two-year-old Bloodhound who exhibits coughing, shallow breathing, generalized malaise, and uveitis (93a). Aspiration of the vitreous reveals the cytology shown (93b).
i. What organism is depicted in 93b?
ii. Describe the pathophysiology of this disease.
iii. What is the treatment?

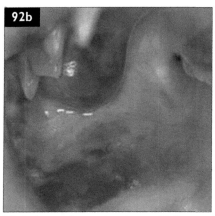

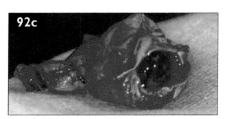

92 i. An oral examination, which revealed a swelling behind the last molar (92b). Pain on opening the mouth suggests an orbital inflammatory disease. No pain on opening the mouth indicates the possibility of a noninflammatory neoplastic disease. Examination of the oral cavity near the last molar for abnormal swellings, discharge, and dental disease can help with diagnosis. If there is swelling, exploration is indicated after diagnostic imaging. Orbital abscesses can be drained from the area posterior to the last molar (see cases 9, 146, and 166). Culture, cytology, biopsy, and molar extraction may all be indicated.
ii. This was a case of orbital invasion of a sinus lymphoma. The globe was enucleated in an to attempt to save the cat's life (92c). Radiation/chemotherapy can be instigated for the sinus tumor.

93 i. *Blastomyces dermatitidis*, a dimorphic fungus that causes canine blasto-mycosis.
ii. *B. dermatitidis* is not transmitted between animals, but rather is acquired by inhalation of the spores. Dissemination of the fungus through the blood and lymph results in a generalized, multisystemic, pyogranulomatous disease. Approximately 30–40% of dogs who acquire the disease will also develop ocular signs. The most common manifestations are pyogranulomatous inflammation of the anterior and posterior segment, with secondary glaucoma and retinal detachment. However, clinically, uveitis is most commonly diagnosed.
iii. The currently recommended treatment is systemic itraconazole for up to three months. Topical corticosteroids and mydriatic agents are required to control the uveitis until infection has been resolved. Secondary glaucoma can develop.

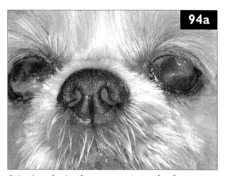
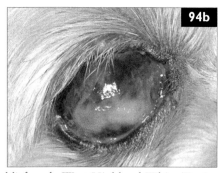

94 A relatively young (nearly four-year-old) female West Highland White Terrier was presented in the clinic with a copious mucoid to mucopurulent discharge covering the corneas of both eyes (**94a, b**). In addition, the dog was exhibiting blepharospasm and conjunctivitis. The corneas appeared dull, with some neovascularization and pigmentation. The Schirmer tear test reading was 4 mm wetting/minute in each eye. The owners had been frequently complaining to their veterinarian of 'chronic eye infection'. While topical medication had provided improvement in the past, the problem was never resolved.
i. What is the most likely cause for this dog's eye condition?
ii. What can be done to resolve this condition medically?
iii. What can be done to resolve this condition surgically?

95 A seven-year-old domestic short-haired cat is presented with decreased vision. On ophthalmoscopic examination there are linear tracks across the retina (**95**).
i. What are the differentials for this condition?
ii. What is the most common etiology of this condition?
iii. What are the treatment options?

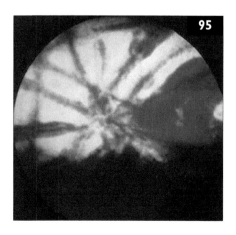

94 i. Keratoconjunctivitis sicca (KCS). West Highland White Terriers are at risk of KCS and thus this dog's KCS is probably breed related.

ii. Up to four months of medical treatment should always be attempted, as the lacrimal gland can take that long to repair itself once medical therapy is initiated. The goals of KCS therapy are to remove pain and maintain vision. First, replace tears with artificial tear replacers. Serum can also be used as tear replacement therapy. Second, stimulate the production of tears with topical 0.2% cyclosporin A (CSA) BID. CSA is known to inhibit T lymphocyte-induced apoptosis of lacrimal gland acinar cells and to reduce adenitis. It interferes with prolactin, has anti-inflammatory activity, and greatly reduces pigmentary/inflammatory keratitis. Topical 0.03% tacrolimus and 1% pimecrolimus (both BID) have similar immunomodulating effects to CSA and may also be used. Oral 2% pilocarpine (1 drop/10 kg BID) also can be effective in neurogenic cases of KCS. Third, corneal infection and keratitis should be reduced with topical broad-spectrum antibiotic (BID) and topical corticosteroid (but not if corneal ulcerations are present).

iii. A conjunctival flap should be constructed in order to provide corrective tissue and blood vessels to any deep corneal ulcers. In patients who do not respond to medical therapy and/or patients whose owners cannot manage medical therapy, transposition of the parotid duct could be performed. Note that saliva is not a perfect tear substitute, but is adequate in most cases.

95 i. The presence of arcuate or linear depigmented areas in the feline fundus may be due to traumatic, degenerative, or inflammatory disease of the retinal pigment epithelium. Curvilinear tracts in the ocular fundus of cats have been associated with the presence of parasitic insect larval stages and are termed ophthalmomyiasis interna posterior. Clinical findings are usually incidental. Curvilinear tracks are present in the tapetal as well as the nontapetal fundus.

ii. Ophthalmomyiasis is rare in cats. *Cuterebra* larvae are the most often reported cause of feline ophthalmomyiasis. The parasite migrates in and around the sensory retina. Most affected cats are asymptomatic, but some can have signs of anterior uveitis.

iii. The treatment of choice for inflamed eyes is systemic corticosteroids. Topical anti-inflammatories should be given to patients with anterior uveitis. Rarely, the larva can be seen in the anterior chamber or vitreous, and surgical extraction may be recommended.

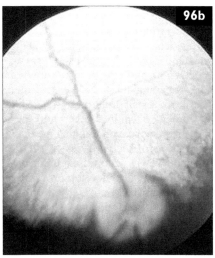

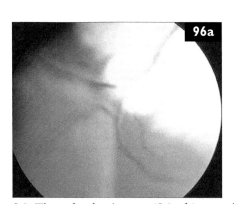

96 These fundus images (96a, b) are taken from a four-year-old Samoyed that presented with blindness, mild iris color change, and depigmentation of the nasal planum.
i. What is the cause of the blindness?
ii. What is the most likely diagnosis considering the breed and clinical signs?
iii. What is the treatment?

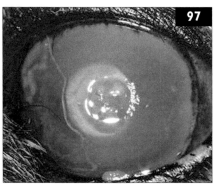

97 A seven-year-old mixed breed dog was presented with a deep melting stromal corneal ulcer (97). The medical term for 'melting' is keratomalacia. What is the mechanism for the 'melting' process, and how is it manifest clinically?

96 i. Bullous retinal detachment (191a).
ii. The retinal detachment, iris color
change from uveitis, nose depigmentation, and breed suggest uveodermatologic syndrome (UVD), also known as
Vogt–Koyanagi–Harada-like syndrome.
The most recent hypothesis regarding
the etiology of canine UVD syndrome is
that it results from an immune-mediated
destruction of melanocytes of the eye
and skin. The iris and retinal pigmented
epithelium can also develop progressive

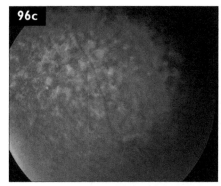

depigmentation (96c). Dermal and hair depigmentation (vitiligo and poliosis,
respectively) develop. The lesions are usually restricted to the face, involving the
eyelids, nasal planum, and lips, but the scrotum and footpads are other areas of
possible dermal involvement (see case 3).
iii. Initial therapy involves immunosuppressive doses of oral prednisone ±
azathioprine or cyclophosphamide. Azathioprine has a lag period of 3–5 weeks
before it becomes effective, therefore tapering of corticosteroids should not be
attempted before this period. Maintenance therapy may require one or both drugs
at a markedly reduced dose. Topical corticosteroids may be used for anterior
segment lesions. The prognosis for dogs affected with UVD syndrome is guarded,
and therapy should be considered to be lifelong. Relapses are frequent if therapy is
stopped or tapered.

97 Keratomalacia, or 'melting', is corneal stromal collagen dissolution and
liquefaction under the influence of elevated levels of tissue, microbial, and tear film
proteases. The keratomalacia gives a grayish-gelatinous liquefied appearance to the
ulcer and the ulcer margin. Melting stroma in the early stages may be difficult to
distinguish from corneal edema. This catastrophic corneal degenerative condition
may deteriorate rapidly and lead to corneal perforation and iris prolapse in as few
as 12–48 hours. Proteolytic enzymes (proteases) perform important physiologic
functions in the normally slow turnover and remodeling of the corneal stroma.
Natural protease inhibitors are also present in the precorneal tear film and in the
cornea. These normally prevent excessive degradation of normal healthy tissue.
Melting corneal disorders occur when there is an imbalance between proteases and
protease inhibitors in favor of the proteases, therefore causing pathologic
degradation of stromal collagen and proteoglycans in the cornea.

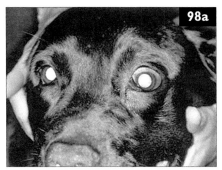

98 A nine-year-old female Labrador Retriever is presented with a two-week history of progressive enlargement of her left eye (98a).
i. Is the dog buphthalmic or exophthalmic? What diagnostic tests will be helpful?
ii. What are the major differentials?
iii. What diagnostic test should be performed?
iv. What are the options for therapy?

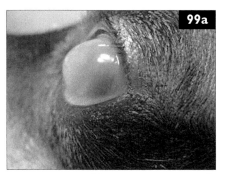
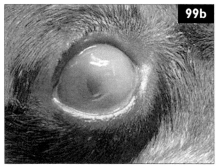

99 A six-year-old cat is presented with rapid onset of the bulging, cloudy corneal disease seen in 99a, b. No known trauma is reported, but the cat does go outdoors during the day. There is no fluorescein dye retention.
i. What are your differential diagnoses?
ii. What is the most likely diagnosis?
iii. What is the pathophysiology of the disease?
iv. What treatment is recommended?

98 i. A high intraocular pressure (IOP) indicates glaucoma and possible buphthalmos. On retropulsion of both eyes, a buphthalmic eye will retropulse well and an exophthalmic eye will retropulse with difficulty (see cases **9, 101,** and **166**). Pain on opening the mouth indicates extraocular inflammation (see case **146**). Measuring the horizontal corneal diameters can also aid differentiation of the enlarged globe of buphthalmos compared with the normal globe in exophthalmos. This dog has normal IOPs, poor retropulsion, and no pain on opening the mouth, indicating that the

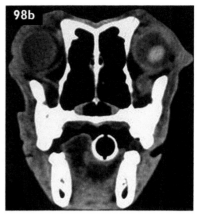

patient is exophthalmic, with a possible orbital mass as the cause.
ii. Orbital abscess, orbital cellulitis, orbital emphysema, orbital hematoma, orbital pseudotumor, orbital tumor, extraorbital tumor (sinus or nasal), and trauma.
iii. Diagnostic imaging. Ocular ultrasound is a reliable way of examining the orbit. Advanced imaging (CT, MRI) is best for determining the extent of tissue invasion and is helpful for surgical plans (**98b,** CT of the dog reveals an optic nerve meningioma).
iv. Small tumors not involving the optic nerve may be removed surgically with orbitotomy to keep a visual eye. Most patients require an extenteration for orbital tumors.

99 i. Differentials include descemetocele, corneal foreign body, iris prolapse, corneal epithelial inclusion cyst, acute bullous keratopathy, and corneal endothelial dystrophy.
ii. A large corneal bulla is present and the cornea appears soft (**99b**). The diagnosis is acute bullous keratopathy.
iii. Acute onset of corneal edema due to a possible stromal defect leads to formation of small vesicles in the corneal epithelium that coalesce into larger bullae, which may rupture, causing loss of epithelium and corneal ulceration. The condition resembles a melting ulcer, but has an acute onset.
iv. Treatment requires support be provided to the cornea by a nictitans flap and/or possibly a tarsorrhaphy to reduce the chance of bullae rupturing. Topical antibiotics, 1% atropine, 5% topical hypertonic NaCl ointment or solution, and antiprotease treatment with autologous serum are recommended. A conjunctival flap is also indicated for many cases of bullous keratopathy.

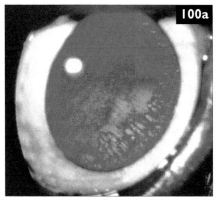

100 A five-year-old female Siberian Husky with diabetes mellitus was presented for her annual examination. A general physical examination was performed. Ophthalmology examination with pharmacologic mydriasis revealed the finding shown (100a).
i. Describe the lenticular changes in this dog.
ii. What is the mechanism by which diabetes mellitus induces these lens changes?
iii. What stage of lens disease is present?

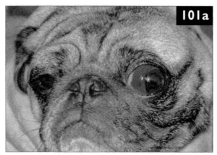

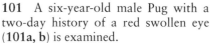

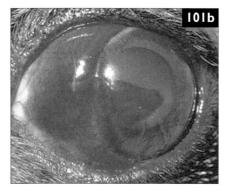

101 A six-year-old male Pug with a two-day history of a red swollen eye (101a, b) is examined.
i. Describe the lesion.
ii. What are the diagnosis and etiology?
iii. What is the treatment?
iv. What is the prognosis for vision?

100 i. Early cataractous changes are observed in the form of equatorial cortical vacuoles. Note the red fundic reflection in this dog due to the lack of the tapetum (which is consistent with its blue iris and light coat color).

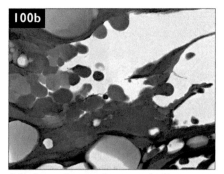

ii. Glucose is the main lens energy source. Lens hexokinase normally converts glucose to glucose-6-phosphate, but is overwhelmed by the excess levels of glucose in the diabetic lens. Aldose reductase normally only metabolizes 5% of the lens glucose, but metabolizes up to 33% of the excess glucose to sorbitol in the diabetic lens. Sorbitol dehydrogenase (SD) normally breaks down sorbitol to fructose, but SD is overwhelmed in diabetics and sorbitol thus accumulates in the lens. The sorbitol osmotically draws water into the lens, causing lens fiber swelling and rupture. These early cataractous changes appear as vacuoles in the equatorial lens cortex in dogs and may be seen in the posterior cortex of diabetic cats. Diabetic cataracts rapidly progress to maturity in dogs (**100b**).

iii. The cataracts in this dog are incipient. Incipient cataract refers to early clinically apparent cataractous changes involving less than 15% of the lens volume.

101 i. The right eye is swollen and rostrally displaced in the orbit. There is dark red scleral hemorrhage, lateral strabismus, and some corneal pigmentation.

ii. Proptosis, a forward displacement of the eye from the orbit seen commonly with retrobulbar hemorrhage and edema following trauma. Often, there is sufficient trauma to cause stretching and/or tearing of extraocular muscles. Proptosis occurs fairly commonly in dogs (especially brachycephalics).

iii. The eye should be kept moist pre-surgically. This is something the owner can do on the way to the emergency clinic. A temporary tarsorrhaphy is performed under general anesthesia and the sutures are kept in place for 1–3 weeks. Medical treatment with systemic antibiotics and topical antibiotic ointment and atropine is indicated. Systemic anti-inflammatory drugs may be used to help decrease severe swelling of the periocular tissue.

iv. Proptosed eyes should be evaluated for hyphema, pupillary light reflexes, and extraocular muscle damage. All proptosed eyes should be fluorescein stained to evaluate for corneal ulceration. If there are favorable prognostic indicators (absence of hyphema, short duration of proptosis, the muscles intact, the pupil miotic) the eye should be replaced. However, many proptosed eyes do not regain vision.

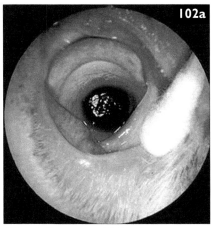
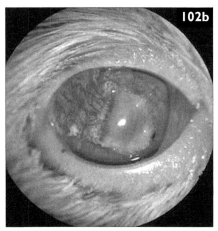

102 A five-year-old Persian cat was presented for an anterior ocular problem (102a).
i. What is your diagnosis?
ii. What is the etiology?
iii. What treatment has been carried out in this cat (102b)?

103 A five-year-old dog is presented for a routine wellness examination. The owner notes that something strange has occurred in the dog's blue eye (103). She is unsure if any trauma could have occurred, but suggests it is unlikely. You draw blood for a complete blood count (CBC) and serum chemistry analysis.
i. What do you expect to find on the CBC based on the ocular changes seen?

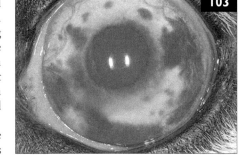

ii. Explain the pathophysiology of this iris condition.
iii. How would you treat this dog, and what is the prognosis?

102 i. Corneal sequestrum, an area of corneal stromal necrosis. Corneal sequestra are usually unilateral and appear as a brown or black, oval to round plaque of the central or paracentral cornea.

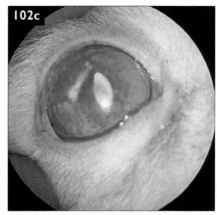

ii. Unknown. However, it is likely due to chronic corneal irritation or previous trauma. Connections between corneal sequestrum and feline herpesvirus, keratoconjunctivitis sicca, nonhealing superficial ulcer, and entropion have been noted. Grid keratectomy of superficial ulcers should not be performed in cats, as it may lead to corneal sequestra. Cats receiving topical or subconjunctival corticosteroids are more likely to develop corneal sequestra, possibly through activation of feline herpesvirus-1.

iii. Superficial keratectomy with corneoscleral transposition. Healthy cornea, limbus, and conjunctiva have been transposed to cover the keratectomy site. Six weeks postoperatively there is good corneal healing, with no recurrence of the sequestrum (**102c**). The transposition site is healed, but the limbal area remains opaque.

103 i. A thrombocytopenia. Causes of thrombocytopenia in dogs include infectious disease (ehrlichiosis, Rocky Mountain spotted fever), neoplasia, and, most commonly, immune-mediated conditions.

ii. Thrombocytopenia in dogs results in a decreased ability to maintain blood homeostasis, therefore hemorrhaging throughout the body and eye is likely. Ocular changes associated with thrombocytopenia include hyphema, petechiation of the iris and sclera, and retinal hemorrhaging. Retinal hemorrhage can result in a disruption in the retinal layers, leading to retinal detachment and blindness.

iii. Treatment depends on the diagnosis. In the case of the more common immune-mediated thrombocytopenia, corticosteroid therapy is effective in controlling the disease. Tetracycline administration for up to one month will combat tick-borne illness-induced thrombocytopenia. Resolution of the thrombocytopenia will reduce any hemorrhaging in the eye. Hyphema is treated with standard uveitic corticosteroid therapy, as in this case. Blindness may still result if retinal detachment has occurred. The prognosis is good if the symptoms can be controlled and if the disease is treated in a timely manner.

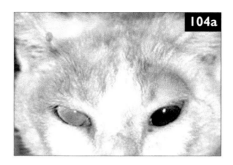
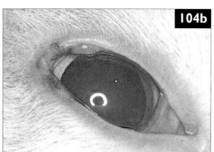

104 A four-year-old cat is presented
with eyelid and conjunctival granulomas
(104a, b). On fundic examination there
is retinitis and a retinal detachment
(104c).
i. What are the major differentials?
ii. What diagnostic test may be helpful
in this case?
iii. What are the endemic areas for this
disease?
iv. What are the treatment options?

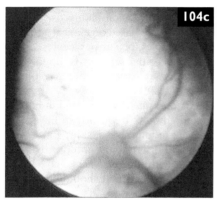

105 A one and a half-year-old Labrador
Retriever is presented with chronic
tearing and redness of the eyes. On
physical examination the right eyelid is
pulled ventrally to demonstrate the
conjunctiva of the third eyelid. You
observe that a small amount of dirt has
collected in the lower eyelid and appears
to be trapped there (105).
i. What is your diagnosis?
ii. What do you tell the owner?
iii. How could you resolve this problem?

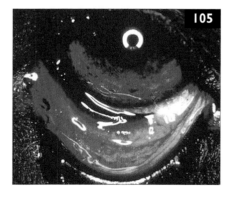

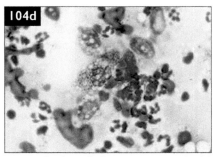

104 i. Systemic mycoses, which include cryptococcosis, histoplasmosis, blasto-mycosis, and coccidioidomycosis (see cases 76 and 186).
ii. Diagnosis is based on clinical and ocular signs, radiographs, stained smears from tissue samples, ocular paracentesis, peripheral lymph node aspirates, culture, and serology. Positive serology is supportive of the diagnosis, but cats with disseminated infection may have negative serology. Cytology identified *Histoplasma* fungus in this cat (104d).
iii. *Histoplasma* is widespread in both North and South America, and is becoming diagnosed more frequently in Europe and Turkey. Common sites for disseminated disease are lung, bone, skin, and visceral organs. Ocular lesions include granulo-matous chorioretinitis, anterior uveitis, retinal detachment, and optic neuritis.
iv. Cats with histoplasmosis have been successfully treated with itraconazole. An internal medicine text should be consulted for current treatment options.

105 i. Persistent conjunctivitis due to medial canthal pocket syndrome.
ii. Medial canthal pocket syndrome is found in large breed dogs such as Rottweilers and Labrador Retrievers. Due to the large orbit in some breeds, a 'pocket' forms at the nasal canthus and collects debris. This debris elicits a focal conjunctivitis of the third eyelid, with the rest of the conjunctiva normal.
iii. Treatment is palliative, as this condition is due to an anatomic problem. Topical steroids and antibiotics can reduce inflammation if severe.

106 A five-year-old male domestic shorthaired cat is presented with a one-week history of third eyelid protrusion (106a).
i. Describe the lesion.
ii. What is the diagnosis, and what is the pathophysiology of this condition?
iii. What are the most common causes of this condition?
iv. What test can be performed to help locate the lesion in this cat?

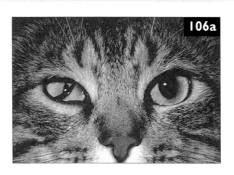

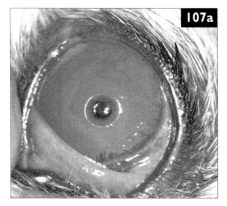

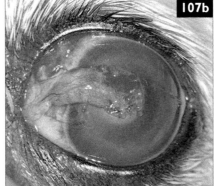

107 A dog is presented with a painful eye. A deep ulcer is present, with slight limbal vascularization and corneal edema (107a). A conjunctival pedicle flap was surgically placed. The eye is shown four days postoperatively (107b).
i. Why was a pedicle flap used rather than a third eyelid flap?
ii. What medications are indicated topically at this point?
iii. This is the eye 40 days post-operatively (107c). What therapy is recommended at this point?

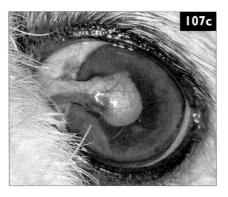

106   i. There is nictitans protrusion, miosis, and ptosis of the right eye.
ii. Horner's syndrome. Loss of adrenergic innervation to Müllers muscle of the upper eyelid results in narrowing of the palpebral fissure and ptosis. Lack of sympathetic tone and enophthalmos results in protrusion of the nictitans. Reduction of normal sympathetic tone to the iris dilator muscle results in miosis in the affected eye. Adrenergic neurons of

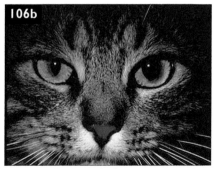

the sympathetic pathway to the eye travel between the hypothalamus and the first three thoracic segments of the spinal cord. A lesion in this part of the pathway produces a first-order Horner's syndrome. Adrenergic neurons then exit the thoracic spinal cord and move in the cranial chest to join the thoracic sympathetic trunk and synapse in the cranial cervical ganglion. A lesion to this neuron will produce a second-order Horner's syndrome. The last neuron in the sympathetic pathway exits the cranial cervical ganglion to innervate the iris dilator muscle. A lesion to this neuron will produce a third-order Horner's syndrome.
iii. Idiopathic, anterior mediastinal neoplasia, otitis media, cervical trauma.
iv. Topical epinephrine 0.001% or phenylephrine 10% should be applied and the time to pupil dilation recorded. If the lesion is postganglionic, the pupil dilates rather quickly (within ~20 minutes), and slower (within ~30–40 minutes) if preganglionic. In this cat the condition resolved 30 minutes after instillation of topical epinephrine (106b). This patient most likely has a preganglionic lesion involving the ear, brachial plexus, or anterior chest.

107   i. A pedicle flap provides physical support to the weakened cornea, a controlled blood supply to the lesion, direct plasma perfusion of antiproteases to the lesion, and fibroblasts to scar the corneal lesion. A third eyelid flap only provides physical support.
ii. Topical antibiotics, atropine, and antiproteases to reduce infection, dilate the pupil, and reduce tear film proteases, respectively.
iii. The flap can be transected to leave a small corneal scar.

108 Bilateral retinal lesions are found in this English Springer Spaniel (108a).
i. Describe the lesions seen.
ii. In what breeds does this retinal problem most commonly occur?
iii. What are some causes of this type of retinal disease?
iv. What is the most likely cause of the specific retinal disease in this English Springer Spaniel?

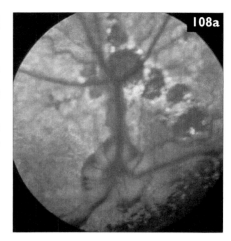

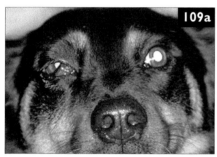

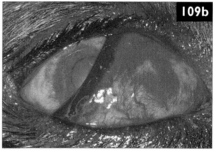

109 An eight-year-old female Rottweiler is brought to the clinic with acute exophthalmos of its right eye (109a, b).
i. What are the clinical signs illustrated?
ii. During the examination, the eye cannot be retropulsed. What are the possible differentials for exophthalmos in this dog?
iii. During the examination the veterinarian attempted to open the mouth of this dog. The dog yelped in pain and twisted his neck and head to move away. What differential moves to the top of the list when pain on opening the mouth is observed?
iv. What is the treatment for this condition?

108 i. There are several medium to large, dark pigmented, irregularly ovoid to circular focal lesions in the tapetum superior to the optic nerve head (ONH) around the dorsal retinal vessels. Areas of hyperreflectivity circumferential to these lesions indicate thinning of the retina at this location. This observation is seen histologically (108b). Dark triangular areas of scleral pigment are

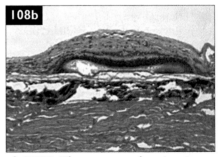

noted in several locations of the peripheral ONH. The nontapetal region is not visible in this photograph. The diagnosis is geographic retinal dysplasia.
ii. Labrador Retrievers and English Springer Spaniels.
iii. Possible causes include heredity, idiopathic, viral infections, vitamin A deficiency, trauma *in utero*, or toxins.
iv. A dominant inheritance with incomplete penetrance.

109 i. There is blepharospasm of the right eye, a miotic pupil, protrusion of the third eyelid, and hyperemia of the conjunctiva of the third eyelid.
ii. Prior to the information included about the inability to retropulse the right eye, Horner's syndrome could have been on the list of differentials as Horner's syndrome also has ptosis, miosis, enophthalmos, and protrusion of the third eyelid (see case 139). The differentials for exophthalmos with conjunctival hyperemia and the inability to retropulse a globe would include orbital cellulitis, retrobulbar abscess (secondary to a tooth root abscess, or foreign material behind the eye), and orbital neoplasia (see case 98).
iii. Retrobulbar abscess or orbital cellulitis.
iv. The abscess is drained by making an incision posterior to the last upper molar on the side of the face with the affected eye (see cases 9, 146, and 166). It is important to be wary of the close proximity to the maxillary artery, optic nerve, and ciliary nerves when entering the retrobulbar space with surgical instruments. The drainage from the abscess should be submitted for aerobic and anaerobic culture. The patient should be placed on oral antibiotics and anti-inflammatories, as well as antibiotic ointment topically on the affected eye. If the exophthalmia is causing exposure of the cornea, a temporary tarsorrhaphy may be indicated.

110 This 18-week-old Persian kitten was presented with a complaint of blindness, having quiet, blind eyes.
i. Describe the funduscopic findings (110).
ii. What is your diagnosis, and what is the etiology?

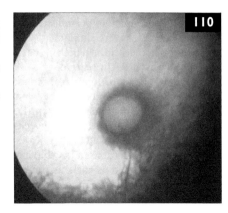

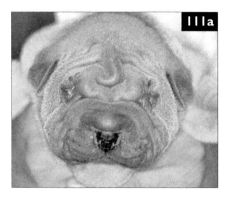

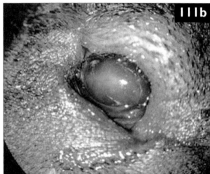

111 A litter of very young (two-week-old) Shar Pei puppies was brought into the clinic with excess forehead skin and severe entropion preventing them from effectively opening their palpebral fissures (111a). Blepharospasm spasticity of the eyelids occurred bilaterally. Close inspection of the corneas reveals some irritation to their anterior surfaces.
i. What are the etiologies of canine entropion?
ii. What temporary corrective measures have been used in this Shar Pei (111b, c)?

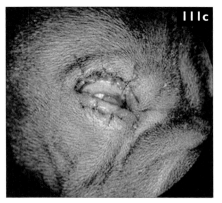

110 i. There is tapetal hyperreflectivity, retinal vessels attenuation, and optic nerve atrophy. Both eyes were similar.

ii. Retinal degeneration, which in cats can be genetic (often termed progressive retinal atrophy [PRA]), secondary to inflammatory retinal or choroidal diseases, drug induced (e.g. enrofloxacin), secondary to taurine deficiency, or associated with previous retinal detachment. In the Persian cat, an autosomal recessive, progressive retinal degeneration has been identified. The earliest clinical sign is a reduced pupillary light reflex noted at 2–3 weeks of age. By 16 weeks, retinal degeneration is complete. The Siamese breed is also at risk, but all cat breeds can be potentially affected. Abyssinian cats can develop a form of PRA called rod-cone dysplasia, with kittens being affected as early as four weeks of age. A rod-cone degeneration can also form in the Abyssinian as a second form of progressive retinal degeneration. This does not begin until 1.5–2 years of age and progresses to complete degeneration in 2–4 years. The ophthalmoscopic findings can be confirmed on electroretinography. Unfortunately, treatment is not available for this condition and these diseases.

111 i. Entropion may result from a difference in tension between the orbicularis oculi muscle and the malaris muscle (lower lid entropion), and is influenced by multiple conditions such as the length of the lid fissure, conformation of the skull, the orbital anatomy, gender, and the extensiveness of folds of the facial skin around the eye. Entropion in the dog occurs either as a developmental anatomic problem or secondarily as an acquired condition due to other ongoing lid, orbital, conjunctival, corneal, intraocular, or systemic disease processes. Many breeds have a predisposition to entropion. The condition is particularly common in the Shar Pei, where it can be severe, affecting pups as early as 14 days of age, as in this case. In large breeds (e.g. Bull Mastiff, Doberman Pinscher, Great Dane, Rottweiler) the large orbit size and/or macropalpebral fissure can also contribute to inadequate lid support resulting in entropion.

ii. Tacking of the affected eyelids with mattress sutures. Staples could have been used. Before surgery can be performed the degree of lid spasticity exacerbating the amount of anatomic entropion must be determined with topical anesthesia in an awake dog, There are various surgical treatments for the permanent correction of entropion in dogs older than six months of age and in adult dogs. The most common treatment involves the Hotz–Celsus surgical technique.

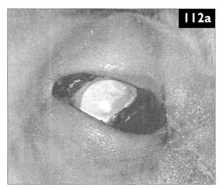

112 A 13-year-old cat is seen with a three-week history of a swollen red eye (**112a**).
i. Describe the lesion.
ii. What are the differentials?
iii. What test should be performed?
iv. What are the treatment options?

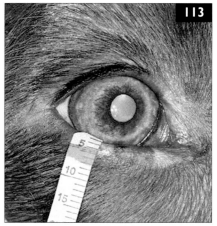

113 The Schirmer tear test (STT) is a tool for assessing ophthalmic-associated tissues (**113**).
i. What does the STT assess?
ii. How long should the test be performed?
iii. What are the normal STT values?

112 i. There is severe periocular swelling and exophthalmos. The pupil is dilated and there is hyperemic conjunctivitis with chemosis.

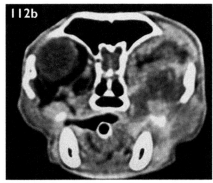

ii. Differentials include orbital abscess, orbital cellulitis, orbital emphysema, orbital pseudotumor, orbital tumor, extraorbital tumor (sinus or nasal), and trauma.

iii. Diagnostic imaging and an oral examination (see cases 92, 220, and 254) should be performed in all cases of progressive exophthalmos. Skull radiographs and orbital ultrasound may be helpful in the diagnosis of orbital abscess, orbital cellulitis, orbital trauma (foreign body), and orbital emphysema. In patients with orbital tumors, advanced imaging is helpful for surgical planning. CT was used to delineate the borders of this tumor (112b).

iv. Surgery may only be a palliative therapy because 90% of feline orbital neoplasms are malignant. The therapy of choice for most orbital tumors is enucleation or exenteration.

113 i. The aqueous layer of the precorneal tear film is evaluated quantitatively by the STT. The diagnosis of 'dry eye' (keratoconjunctivitis [KCS]) may be missed if the STT is not routinely used. Topical anesthesia and other eye drops are avoided before the test. The round end of the test paper is bent while still in the envelope and positioned without contamination in the lacrimal lake at the junction of the lateral and middle third of the lower eyelid. The animal usually closes its eyelids during the test.

ii. The STT strip should be left in position for one minute. It is not a linear test, so if you obtain a value of 7 mm/30 seconds, this does not mean it will be 14 mm/minute. The first 30 seconds of the STT are faster then the last 30 seconds.

iii. Dog, 21.9 ± 4.0 mm wetting/minute; cat, 20.2 ± 4.5 mm wetting/minute. Dogs with slightly lower than normal STT values are suspicious for dry eye if the STT value is combined with clinical signs (dry corneal surface, corneal visualization, corneal pigmentation, conjunctival hyperemia, mucoid ocular discharge, blepharospasm). STT values <5 mm/minute are diagnostic for dry eye (KCS) in dogs. STT values in a normal cat can be 5 mm/minute with no clinical signs, but a low STT value with concurrent clinical signs is diagnostic for feline KCS.

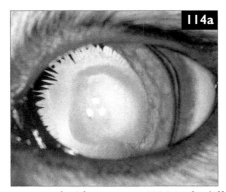

114 An adult cat was presented with a cataract (114a) of a different type to the one seen in case 51.
i. What are the dark, finger-like projections noted from about eight to 12 o'clock?
ii. What type of cataract is depicted in 114a?
iii. What secondary clinical signs might be noted on examination of a cat with this type of cataract?

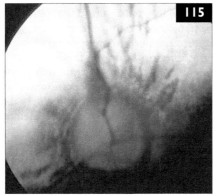

115 This ophthalmoscopic examination (115) was performed in a dog four weeks post proptosis of the globe. Findings included optic nerve head (ONH) atrophy with blood vessels attenuation and retinal nerve fiber layer hemorrhages. The intraocular pressure was normal.
i. What is the pathophysiology of these findings?
ii. What is the most likely diagnosis?

114 i. Pigmented ciliary body processes. The lens zonules arise from these
ciliary processes and attach at the lens
equator to suspend the lens in position.
ii. A resorbing hypermature cataract.
Hypermature cataracts are associated
with a reduction in lens volume, a
wrinkled lens capsule (**114b**, histological
image from a plastic section of a
resorbing cataract), an increased ability

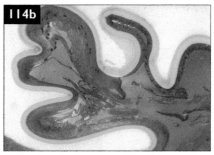

to visualize the tapetal reflection due to a reduction in lens opacification, and an
increase in the depth of the anterior chamber. The reduction in lens volume during
the resorption of a hypermature cataract causes the lens capsule to contract and
pull on the lens zonules, and thus stretch the ciliary processes. This is the reason
why the ciliary processes are so visible in this eye. Anterior uveitis can also be noted
with rapidly forming and hypermature cataracts.
iii. Clinical signs associated with anterior uveitis (e.g. flare, synechiae, rubeosis
iridis) may be noted when evaluating a cat with a resorbing hypermature
cataract. Leakage of lens proteins through the intact lens capsule initiates an
inflammatory uveitic reaction, as these proteins are not recognized as self by the
eye's immune system.

115 i. All portions of the optic nerve (i.e. intraocular, intraorbital, intracanalicular,
intracranial) are susceptible to traumatic injury from head trauma. Force applied to
the anterior orbit can be transmitted to the optic foramen, with subsequent traction,
contusion, and shearing forces applied to the optic nerve and small nutrient vessels.
Rapid deceleration of the anterior portion of the optic nerve relative to the fixed
posterior portion of the canine optic nerve in traumatic globe proptosis can cause
ONH avulsion, globe rupture, optic nerve laceration and atrophy, and vascular
compromise to the ONH. Hemorrhage after trauma may disrupt the optic nerve
parenchyma or accumulate within the nerve sheaths. Hemorrhage into the optic
nerve or interference with its blood supply as the result of trauma can also result
in optic nerve vascular compromise as a consequence of short posterior ciliary
artery vessel thrombosis and subsequent ischemia. Intracanalicular optic nerve
trauma can result from direct damage by penetrating foreign bodies, compression,
and orbital bone fractures, or it can result from a blow to the frontal region.
ii. Traumatic optic nerve atrophy. A number of treatment options have been
advocated, including systemic hyperosmotic agents and systemic corticosteroids.
Visual reconvery is not possible in dogs with optic atrophy.

116 A nine-year-old female spayed Boston Terrier is presented with a progressive six-week history of blue eyes (116a). The intraocular pressure is 15 mmHg in both eyes.
i. What is the most likely diagnosis?
ii. Which breeds are most likely to have this disease?
iii. What is the pathology of this condition?
iv. What are the treatment options?

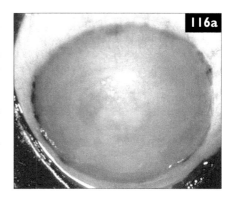

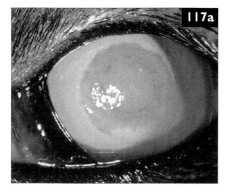

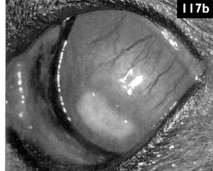

117 A six-year-old Greyhound dog is presented with this corneal ulcer (117a). Therapy consisted of topical antifungals, antibiotics, atropine, and serum.
i. Describe the lesion. Cytology revealed hyphae.
ii. What is the status of healing after four weeks of therapy (117b)?
iii. What is the status of the eye six weeks after therapy was initiated (117c)?

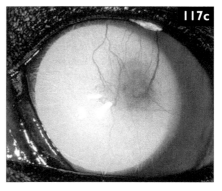

116 i. Corneal edema, which in this case has been caused by endothelial dystrophy. The lack of corneal vascularization and conjunctival hyperemia, and the normal IOPs, rule out uveitis, glaucoma, anterior lens luxation (see case **34**), and corneal ulceration. A slit lamp examination (**116b**) would show the cornea to be 3–5 times thicker than a normal cornea (see case **24** for comparison).

ii. Boston Terrier, Chihuahua, and Dachshund.

iii. Endothelial dystrophy is a progressive, bilateral degeneration of corneal endothelial cells that results in an edematous, avascular cornea. The dystrophic endothelium has a decreased number of cells and exhibits fibrous metaplasia. As the cell layer thins, the fluid pumps of the endothelium cannot keep up with the demand and aqueous humor leaks into the stroma to result in edema.

iv. Topical 5% sodium chloride can pull fluid osmotically out of the cornea and reduce edema in the early stages of disease. When medical therapy fails, a thermokeratoplasty (see case **242**), a Gundersen conjunctival flap, or a full-thickness corneal transplant is recommended. A penetrating keratoplasty with fresh, healthy canine cornea gives the best long-term results (**116c**).

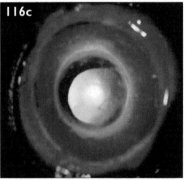

117 i. A white cellular infiltrate with a brown ring is present. The infiltrate is large and involves the superficial and deep cornea. There is little to no corneal vascularization, as is typical for fungal ulcers. The pupil is dilated from a mydriatic.

ii. The corneal fungal plaque is smaller and being invaded by blood vessels. The cornea is healing and remodeling behind the blood vessels. This is a good response.

iii. The ulcer has healed, leaving a small scar. The pupil remains dilated temporally. No therapy is necessary at this time.

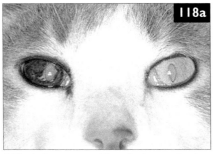
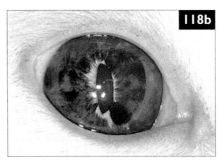

118 A four-year-old male domestic shorthaired cat is presented with an eight-week history of iris color change in his right eye (**118a, b**).
i. What are the differentials for iris color change?
ii. What is the treatment of choice?

119 A six-year-old Irish Setter was presented with the neurophthalmic signs seen in **119a** including ptosis of the lateral two-thirds or so of the right upper eyelid, mydriasis, decreased corneal sensation, reduced globe motility, and slight strabismus (**119b**).
i. What is the most likely cause of this dog's neurophthalmic condition?
ii. What diagnostics can be performed to help determine the location of the lesion?

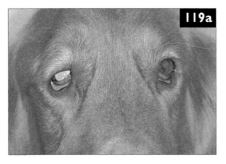
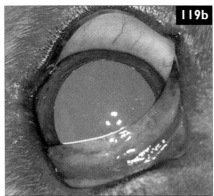

118 i. Uveitis, neoplasia, melanosis.
ii. There is no treatment for iris
melanosis. Monitoring pigment changes
and intraocular pressures every six
months is recommended. Glaucoma can
occur if the iridocorneal angle is
obstructed by pigment. Gonioscopy is
used to determine if the pigment has
migrated into the angle. Ocular ultrasound may be helpful to determine if the
pigment involves more than just the
anterior face of the iris.

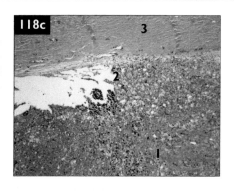

The treatment for diffuse iris melanoma is enucleation. The time to enucleate an
eye will vary according to the progression of diffuse iridal melanoma, and will differ
from individual to individual. Most progress slowly. The presence of tumor cells
within the aqueous outflow pathway greatly increases the likelihood of glaucoma
and of metastasis to the liver and the lung. A micrograph taken from a cat with
iridal melanoma that had progressed to the base of the iris (1) is shown (118c).
Although the tumor cells had not entered the iridocorneal angle (2) or the sclera (3),
the situation certainly was precarious in that case.

119 i. In dogs the oculomotor nerve (CN III), the trochlear nerve (CN IV), the
abducens nerve (CN VI), and the mandibular and ophthalmic branches of the
trigeminal nerve (CN V) all course together through the cavernous sinus and enter
the orbit through the orbital fissure. Clinical signs noted with cavernous sinus
syndrome are associated with dysfunction to these nerves and are collectively
termed ophthalmoplegia. Inability to rotate the globe medially, dorsally, or
ventrally, ptosis, lateral strabismus, decreased corneal sensitivity, possible decreased
or absent corneal blink reflex, and the inability to retract the eye are noted in
external ophthalmoplegia. Lesions to the oculomotor nerve fibers in the cavernous
sinus that cause a dilated pupil that is unable to constrict by either the direct or
indirect pupillary light reflexes are found with internal ophthalmoplegia. The
consensual response from the affected eye to the unaffected is, however, present as
the optic nerve is not affected in cavernous sinus syndrome.
ii. CT and MRI can aid the diagnosis and localization of this neurophthalmic
problem. Trauma and tumors are causes of cavernous sinus syndrome in dogs and
cats.

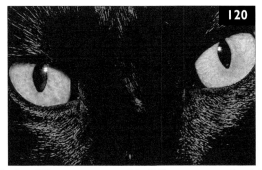

120 An adult black DSH cat presents with different appearing irides (120).
i. How does the right eye differ from the left?
ii. What is the most likely cause of this change in this cat?
iii. What are the possible etiologies for this condition?
iv. Is there a treatment? Will the changes in the right eye resolve with treatment?

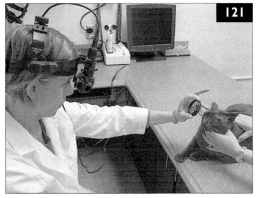

121 Methods to examine the eyes of small animals involve the use of an ophthal-moscope and, in the instance seen here (121), a hand lens in conjunction with a head-set (i.e. indirect ophthalmoscopy).
i. What are the advantages of performing indirect ophthalmoscopy along with direct ophthalmoscopy?
ii. How does one perform indirect ophthalmoscopy effectively?

120 i. The right eye exhibits iris color change. Small, dark foci are present in the iris of the right eye compared with the left.
ii. Uveitis in cats can cause a color change to the iris and other clinical signs (see case 7). Clinical signs with feline uveitis include decreased vision, blepharospasm, corneal edema, aqueous flare, fibrin-filled anterior chamber, hypopyon, anterior vitreal infiltrate, miosis, and iridal hyperemia.
iii. Causes of uveitis in cats include feline immunodeficiency virus, feline infectious peritonitis, feline leukemia virus, fungal infection, toxoplasmosis, and bartonellosis (cases **4**, **177**, and **189**). Trauma, neoplasia, cataracts, and lens luxation are also causes of uveitis in cats (cases **25**, **148**, and **178**).
iv. Therapy for feline uveitis involves suppressing the inflammation with corticosteroid therapy and dilating the pupil with mydriatics. Changes to the iris color from uveitis are unlikely to resolve.

121 i. The advantages of binocular indirect ophthalmoscopy are penetration of cloudy media, large field of view, examination of the peripheral fundus, ease of compensation of refractive errors and eye movements, stereopsis, greater distance between examiner and patient, 2–3 simultaneous observers, and the ability to examine more intractable patients with less hazard to the examiner. The disadvantages include less magnification for studying particular areas and the need for drug-induced mydriasis.
ii. A fairly bright light source is directed into the eye. A condensing lens is interposed between the light source and the eye. Incident light is condensed to illuminate the fundus. The reflected light then is condensed by the same lens to form a virtual, inverted, and reversed image between the lens and the light source. Indirect ophthalmoscopy can be employed with only a light source and a lens. The indirect ophthalmoscope is adjusted so that the light is slightly off center of the examiner's visual field (to reduce glare). The patient's muzzle is held gently and the lens is positioned 3–5 cm from the cornea and the upper eyelid retracted. The lens is usually held close to the cornea initially to permit observation of the ocular fundus and then moved away from the eye until the image is maximum size. When the hand lens is interposed between the light source and the eye, the fundus is visualized. Image magnification (2× to 4×) is dependent on the diopter power of the hand lens. Occasionally, a hindering light reflection may occur and can be remedied by slightly tilting the hand lens.

122 A four-month-old mixed breed puppy is presented with a brown spot on the right eye (122).
i. Describe the lesion.
ii. How does this occur?
iii. What are the treatment options?
iv. In what breeds might this condition be inherited?

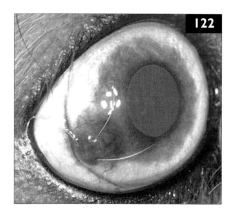

123 Glaucoma insidiously causes damage to the retina and the optic disk and can result in partial to complete blindness without therapeutic intervention.
i. What can be seen in the fundus image (123a) and the scanning electron micrograph (SEM) of a trypsin-digested optic disk (123b) in this dog?
ii. What is the pathologic process present in the glaucomatous optic disk, and what is its significance to saving sight?

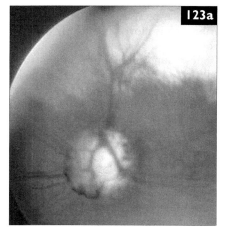

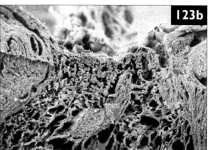

122 i. There is a circular, brown, pigmented, raised, corneal lesion associated with the lateral limbus that has white hairs. This is an example of a corneal dermoid.
ii. A dermoid forms by abnormal invagination of ectodermal tissue during gestation and results in well-differentiated normal tissue in an abnormal location. Histologically, corneal dermoids contain many types of tissue, including glands and cartilage.
iii. Surgery is often required to remove the dermoid; a superficial keratectomy is the best option. The cornea is thin under a dermoid and an operating microscope is recommended for surgical removal.
iv. This congenital condition may be familial or breed-related in Dachshunds, Dalmatians, Doberman Pinschers, German Shepherd Dogs, and St. Bernards, as well as in the Burmese cat.

123 i. Posterior displacement of the optic nerve and scleral lamina cribrosa or optic disk 'cupping' from glaucoma. The round optic nerve head (ONH) is out of focus at the plane of the retinal vessels and focused deeper in the vessels of the center of the optic disk. This is due to posterior movement of the disc in response to elevated intraocular pressure (IOP). All neural tissue is absent in the SEM. The scleral lamina cribrosa has moved posteriorly due to elevated IOP to form the 'optic nerve cup' noted with the ophthalmoscope in advanced canine glaucoma. The SEM demonstrates compression of laminar pores and illustrates the difficulty optic axons would have passing through those pores in glaucoma.
ii. The sclera is a strong and elastic fibrous tissue, but with abrupt and prolonged elevation of IOP it develops functional and anatomic alterations to its collagen and elastin fibers. The specialized region of the sclera through which the optic nerve axons and ocular blood vessels penetrate is termed the scleral lamina cribrosa. This is distorted and compressed posteriorly by increases in IOP, thus affecting axoplasmic flow within the axons and reducing the blood supply to the ONH. The cupping of the ONH associated with glaucoma results from optic nerve axonal death as well as from compression, stretching, and rearrangement of connective tissue of the lamina cribrosa in response to this altered IOP. As damage to the ONH and optic nerve axons progresses, the clinical signs of mydriasis and visual impairment occur.

124 This four-month-old Shih Tzu was born with the problem shown (**124**).
i. What ophthalmic condition does this young dog have?
ii. What are the consequences of the disease?

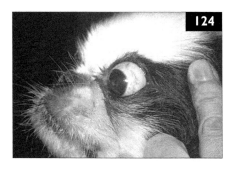

125 This is a funduscopic picture of a kitten with the condition known as lipemia retinalis (**125**). What is lipemia retinalis, and what is its significance?

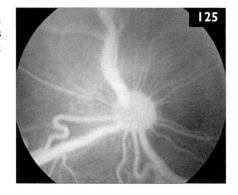

126 A five-year-old German Shepherd Dog was treated with trimethoprim–sulfamethoxazole for urinary tract infection. Two weeks after initiation of therapy the dog was presented for an eye problem (**126**).
i. Describe the clinical findings and determine the diagnosis.
ii. What are the possible causes for this dog's eye condition?
iii. What is the therapy?

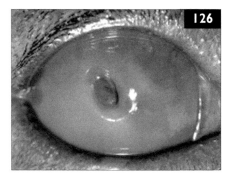

124 i. Euryblepharon or macropalpebral fissure. This is a symmetrical enlargement and widening of the palpebral fissure encountered primarily in brachycephalic dogs with shallow orbits and some large breed dogs. The globe is nearly proptosed in its natural condition to expose a lot of sclera and conjunctiva.
ii. In this dog the condition also resulted in varying degrees of eyelid, blinking, and tear dysfunction. Chronic inflammation of the conjunctiva and corneal irritation can occur. Ophthalmic ointments can protect the cornea in mild cases. Surgical correction with lateral canthoplasty is recommended if corneal disease becomes a problem in dogs with euryblepharon.

125 The term lipemia retinalis describes the ophthalmoscopic visibility of lipids, lipoproteins, or both, in retinal blood vessels. It occurs infrequently in the cat and does not by itself cause retinal pathology. Diseases characterized by defective lipid synthesis or degradation, such as diabetes mellitus, hypothyroidism, and familial hypercholesterolemia due to lipoprotein lipase deficiency, can produce lipemia retinalis. Lipemia retinalis can also be caused by eating a high-lipid diet.

126 i. There is an axial, deep corneal ulcer with diffuse corneal edema and vascularization of the cornea from the dorsal and nasal limbus. The clear, transparent center of the ulcer suggests that this is descemetocele, a type of deep corneal ulcer in which the corneal epithelium and stroma have completely eroded, leaving a corneal lesion lined only by Descemet's membrane and corneal endothelium. When fluorescein stain was applied to the cornea, dye uptake was noted at the corneal stroma exposed at the periphery of the ulcer, but not in the central area, confirming the diagnosis of descemetocele.
ii. Descemetoceles and full-thickness corneal perforation may develop from progression of deep corneal ulcers caused by infection, keratoconjunctivitis sicca (KCS), chemical burns, and trauma. The sulfa component of the systemic antibiotic in this case was toxic to the lacrimal gland and resulted in very low tear production and KCS, which caused the ulcer. Excessive tear film proteases then caused loss of stroma and baring of Descemet's membrane.
iii. Most descemetoceles can be treated successfully using conjunctival grafts or corneal transplantation. Medical therapy should be aggressive and include antiprotease drugs (e.g. serum, EDTA, and N-acetylcysteine), broad-spectrum antibacterial drugs (determined by culture and sensitivity results) topically and systemically, mydriatics (e.g. atropine), and systemically administered NSAIDs.

127 There are instances when clinical signs in an animal indicate an abnormal intraocular pressure (IOP) in one or both eyes. IOP can be assessed by applanation tonometry (127).
i. What are the normal IOP measurements?
ii. What does a low IOP indicate?
iii. What do you do if the tonometer is not working?

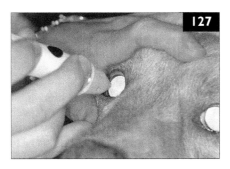

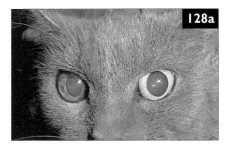

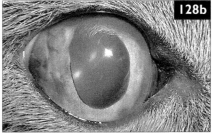

128 Iris color change has taken place in the right eye of this adult cat (128a, b). A large pigmented mass was present and a uveal tumor was diagnosed. The eye was enucleated because of the large size and location of the tumor in the peripheral iris. The enucleated globe was dissected to reveal the extent of tumor invasion (128c).
i. Describe the clinical signs observed in 128a and b.
ii. What is the most likely diagnosis in this adult cat?
iii. Where would the tumor cells that

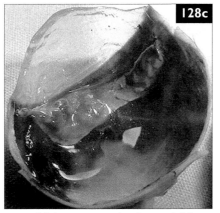

may indicate if metastasis of this tumor could be present be located histopathologically within the eye?
iv. What secondary disease may occur with this type of tumor in its advanced stage?
v. If metastasis occurs, what are two likely locations to which this tumor might spread?
vi. When should the globe be enucleated if this type of tumor is suspected?

125

127 i. Tonometry is an indirect measurement or estimation of IOP. Applanation tonometry measures the force required to flatten a constant area of the cornea. The most popular applanation tonometers, such as the TonoPen, are very accurate and easy to use, and have made it much easier to diagnose animal glaucomas. The normal IOPs are: dogs, 16.8 ± 4.0 mmHg; cats, 20.2 ± 5.5 mmHg

ii. Low IOP, typically <10 mmHg, should raise suspicions of anterior uveitis. Comparison of IOPs in both eyes may be helpful in determining if uveitis is present. Clinical signs of uveitis must also be present to make this diagnosis.

iii. If the TonoPen is not working, first change the TonoPen tip cover and re-calibrate. When the TonoPen reads 'GOOD' you have calibrated the instrument. If the TonoPen reads 'BAD', you have to try again. If TonoPen readings are greater than the 5% error level, then you must try again. Be sure to gently tap the central cornea to get the most accurate readings.

128 i. The iris of the right eye has a color change when compared with the left eye. On closer examination there is a raised, dark tan, thickened, irregularly marginated mass, which is larger laterally than medially. The mass appears to involve the drainage angle. The pupil is dilated and deformed from the nine to 12 o'clock position.

ii. Uveal melanoma.

iii. Tumor cells exfoliate and circulate in the anterior chamber. They then move to the aqueous outflow pathways where they can be found histologically in the filtration meshwork and scleral venous plexus. These cells then have access to the circulation, where they can metastasize.

iv. Secondary glaucoma can occur if the tumor has infiltrated and obstructed a large amount of the drainage angle (see case **118**).

v. Liver and lungs.

vi. Experienced ophthalmologists struggle with this answer as most of these eyes are visual. Enucleation should be recommended if there is aggressive infiltration of the iris, posterior epithelium, or the ciliary body, or if any of the pigmented mass is noted within the iridocorneal angle. The presence of secondary glaucoma is also an indication to enucleate.

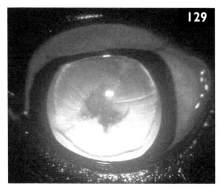

129 This four-month-old Dobermann puppy was presented with microphakia and opacities at the posterior lens capsule (129). There was no history of any eye problem or systemic illness. The pupil was dilated pharmacologically.
i. What is your diagnosis?
ii. What is the etiology of this problem?

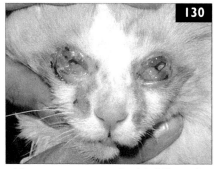

130 A three-month-old cat was presented with bilateral severe blepharospasm, epiphora, mucopurulent discharge, conjunctivitis with chemosis, and symblepharon (130).
i. What is the differential diagnosis?
ii. What diagnostic techniques can be used?
iii. What is the recommended treatment?

129 i. Persistent hyperplasic primary vitreous (PHPV).

ii. The adult lens is avascular, but embryologically the lens has a blood supply known as the tunica vasculosa lentis. The hyaloid artery comprises the primary vitreous and feeds the tunica vasculosa lentis on the posterior part of the lens. In this dog there is apparent proliferation and persistence of the primary vitreous/hyaloid artery/tunica vasculosa lentis tissue known as PHPV instead of the usual atrophy. PHPV is present in young puppies, but may not be noticed until later in life. Clinically, PHPV appears as a white or fibrovascular plaque in the posterior pupil near the posterior lens capsule and anterior vitreous. Vessel ingrowth and frank hemorrhage into the vitreous and lens cortex, calcium deposits, posterior lenticonus, microphakia, lens coloboma, intralental pigmentation, progressive cataracts, and elongated ciliary processes may also be present. Dobermanns and Staffordshire Bull Terriers are predisposed to PHPV.

130 i. Herpesvirus (commonly), calicivirus (rarely), *Chlamydophila*, and, less frequently, *Mycoplasma* are causes of infectious conjunctivitis in cats. Kittens and young cats are most commonly affected. Although herpesvirus and calicivirus are frequently manifested in association with severe upper respiratory tract infections, conjunctivitis may also occur alone.

ii. Virus isolation, indirect fluorescent antibody staining of conjunctival samples, and the demonstration of viral DNA with PCR. The herpesvirus PCR technique is the most sensitive test, although normal, nonsymptomatic cats can give positive results.

iii. Initial treatment for viral keratitis includes 1% trifluridine or 0.1% idoxuridine ophthalmic solutions applied to the affected eye(s) 3–9 times a day. Vidarabine is effective topically, but is sometime difficult to acquire. Cidofovir (0.5%) is effective topically in cats when given BID. Systemic and/or topical alpha-2-interferon (300 U/cat PO SID; 1 drop in affected eye TID or QID) may be beneficial in cats that are refractory to other therapies. Oral famciclovir (62.5 mg/cat SID or BID) for three weeks is effective at reducing herpesvirus clinical signs. Lysine (250–500 mg PO BID) can reduce viral replication in latently infected cats. If corneal ulcerations are present, concurrent treatment with a broad-spectrum topical antibiotic is advised. Antiviral therapy should be continued for 1–2 weeks after resolution of clinical signs. Topical steroids should be used cautiously if at all, as they can increase virus shedding and promote outbreaks of clinical signs in the chronically dormant feline herpes cases.

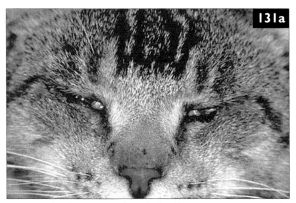

131 A three-year-male domestic shorthaired cat was presented with bilateral entropion (**131a**).
i. What are the causes and clinical signs of entropion in a cat?
ii. What are the treatment options?
iii. Describe the modified Hotz–Celsus procedure.

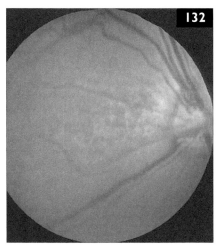

132 This puppy has a small area of choroidal hypoplasia (**132**).
i. What is 'go normal' in relation to Collie eye anomaly (CEA)?
ii. What problems for breeders are associated with the diagnosis of CEA?

131 i. Entropion is an inward rolling of the eyelid margin such that eyelid hairs rub on the cornea. Clinical signs include epiphora, blepharospasm, conjunctivitis, and keratitis. Entropion is uncommon in cats, except for the Persian cat. Feline entropion may be anatomic from microphthalmos, spastic from ocular pain, and cicatricial from scarring.

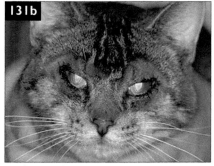

ii. Medical treatment involves using ocular lubricant ointments to protect the cornea from the eyelid hairs. Surgical treatment can be temporary or permanent. Temporary procedures involve using nonabsorbable sutures to evert or 'tack' eyelids in immature animals. When planning and performing permanent entropion surgery, the amount of correction must be estimated prior to general anesthesia. Surgical treatment of entropion should always undercorrect slightly, as postoperative scarring adds to the extent of the correction.

iii. It is a relatively simple procedure that can be adapted to most types of feline entropion (131b). The initial incision is made parallel to and 2–3 mm from the eyelid margin to a depth that includes the orbicularis oculi muscle. The length of the incision is determined by the amount of eyelid margin involved. The ends of the first incision are joined by a ventral elliptical incision, the width previously determined by evaluating the degree of eversion. Closure is with simple interrupted sutures using 4-0 to 6-0 nonabsorbable suture.

132 i. Some Collie dogs have only minor, geographically focal areas of choroidal hypoplasia. These pale areas of choroidal hypoplasia may become masked with pigment as the dog's retina matures. Therefore, by 12 months of age, although genotypically affected, these eyes with focal choroidal hypoplasia may appear clinically normal and are termed 'go-normals'; however, these dogs are still genotypically affected and are carriers for CEA.

ii. Diagnosis of CEA can be made at 4–8 weeks of age. Severely affected puppies can often be identified at this time. Due to the high prevalence in the Collie population, eradication of CEA is very difficult. Breeding minimally affected dogs does not necessarily avoid producing puppies that are severely affected, but it is a practice used by Collie breeders to reduce the prevalence of CEA.

133 A seven-year-old cat is presented with this abnormality (133). The owner informs you that the cat has been on some medication for this eye for 10 months.
i. What do you suspect is wrong with this eye?
ii. What are the etiology and pathophysiology of the condition?
iii. What is a possible complication to the lesions present here?

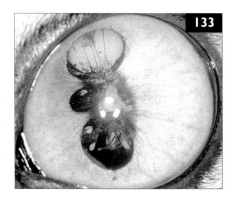

134 This photograph (134) represents a direct ophthalmoscopic view of the fundus of an 11-year-old dog.
i. Describe the clinical signs seen.
ii. What are some possible etiologic diagnoses that may be associated with this condition?
iii. What portion of the retina is affected in this dog?
iv. What diagnostic tests should be performed initially on a patient that presents for this condition?

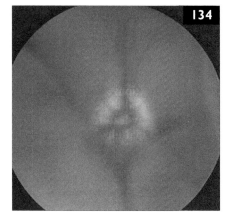

135 The right eye of this cat (135) became suddenly painful. She was squinting and actively pawing at the eye. A foreign body (resting on the holder's finger) was found behind the nictitans in the ventral fornix. What types of ocular damage could be caused by such a wooden foreign body?

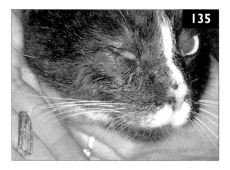

133 i. Posterior synechiae and cataracts have developed secondary to anterior uveitis.

ii. Miosis from the uveitis has increased the normal contact between the lens and iris. Fibrin has caused adhesions between the lens and iris. Iris pigment has migrated on the surface of the lens capsule. The oxidative insult generated by the uveitis has disturbed the lens physiology and resulted in cataract formation.

iii. Posterior synechiae can block aqueous humor movement through the pupil, thus causing glaucoma. The iris bulges anteriorly, which causes scarring and collapse of the iridocorneal angle and a resultant increase in intraocular pressure.

134 i. There are peripheral bullous retinal detachments associated with the ventral fundus. The retinal vessels can be followed onto the anteriorly displaced pillow-like bullous detachments. The borders of the detachment appear distinct.

ii. Possible etiologic diagnoses are infectious (such as tick-borne, bacterial, and mycotic diseases), congenital (such as retinal dysplasia, see case 28), metabolic (such as hypertension, diabetes mellitus, see case 161), neoplastic (such as lymphoma), immune-mediated (such as uveodermatologic syndrome, see cases 3 and 96), and toxin related.

iii. The nine layers of the neurosensory retina are separated from the retinal pigmented epithelium by fluid.

iv. It is important to obtain a complete history, including recent travel, vaccinations, and all medications administered orally. Complete blood count, general chemistry, tick titers, fungal titers, blood pressure, and urinalysis should also be performed. These tests may lead to the necessity of chest and abdominal radiographs as well as an abdominal ultrasound. The retinal detachment in this dog was caused by elevated systemic blood pressure from kidney disease.

135 Superficial corneal ulcers, deep corneal ulcers, and corneal perforation with iris prolapse could occur from an ocular foreign body. The most important factor to evaluate is the integrity of the cornea. Is there an ulcer or has the cornea ruptured? Fluorescein staining and careful evaluation of the anterior chamber depth and pupil size will aid evaluation of the cornea. Infection is also a worry.

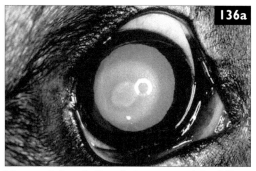

136 A 10-year-old spayed female Beagle is presented for bilateral corneal lesions (136a). The eyes are not painful and the corneas do not retain fluorescein dye.
i. Describe the clinical lesions.
ii. What is the most likely diagnosis?
iii. What are the three morphologic types of this condition that have been described in the literature?
iv. Histologically, what is the make up of these opacities?

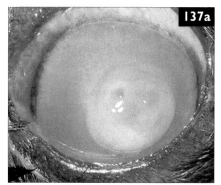
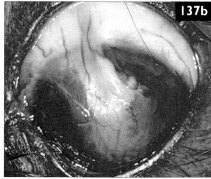

137 A three-and-a-half-year-old mixed breed dog was presented with a melting ulcer and significant corneal stroma loss (137a). The ulcer was treated surgically (137b, three months postoperatively) and medically.
i. What is the pathophysiology of a melting ulcer?
ii. What is the treatment for a melting ulcer, and what is the benefit of a conjunctival or amnion graft?

136 i. A ring-shaped corneal opacity is noted in the paraxial cornea and a second opacity in the center. The smooth flash artifact indicates that these opacities are within the cornea and not the corneal epithelium.

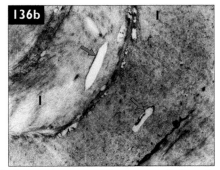

ii. Oval lipid corneal dystrophy in the Beagle dog.

iii. The lesions are located in the subepithelial stroma (compare with case 40). The nebular form of lipid corneal dystrophy is homogeneous with a ground-glass appearance. The racetrack form is a gray oval ring, as seen in this case. It can be located through the entire corneal stroma and is of a more dense opacity than the nebular form. The white arc type is also dense and associated with white plaques of spiculated material.

iv. Cholesterol, neutral fats, and phospholipids are found histologically by frozen sections in lipid corneal dystrophy. Examination by transmission electron microscopy (136b) reveals that the deposits can be crystalline in structure. The deposits (arrows) are randomly placed within the corneal lamellae (1).

137 i. During normal corneal healing, proteases and collagenases are produced that aid in the removal of devitalized cells and debris. Corneal epithelial cells, fibroblasts, polymorphonuclear leukocytes, and microbes produce these enzymes. In some corneal ulcers, overproduction of these enzymes or their reduced inhibition contributes to progressive keratomalacia and rapid 'melting' of the corneal stroma.

ii. Successful management of melting ulcers lies in controlling infection with antibiotics and reducing the impact of enzymatic degradation on the cornea with the help of antiproteases such as serum, EDTA, or N-acetylcysteine. The antiprotease medications (alone or in combination) should be given every 1–2 hours in severe cases. The surgical treatment of choice for fast melting ulcers, however, is a conjunctival flap or amniotic membrane transplant graft. Conjunctival flaps provide a plasma lavage of blood-associated immune components, systemic antibiotics, and natural anticollagenases (e.g. alpha-2-macroglobulin) to the ulcer, provide corneal support to the weakened cornea, provide fibrovascular tissue to fill the corneal defects, and bring a blood supply to the lesion. Amniotic membrane grafts provide massive amounts of antiproteases and physically support the weakened cornea.

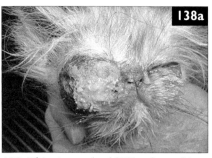
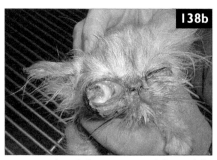

138 This six-week-old Himalayan kitten was rescued and then presented for a right eye problem (138a, b).
i. What is the most likely diagnosis?
ii. What is the material covering the cornea in the first image?
iii. What is the recommended therapy?

139 This four-month-old Irish Setter puppy is presented with a congenital abnormality (139).
i. What is this abnormality?
ii. What is the treatment?

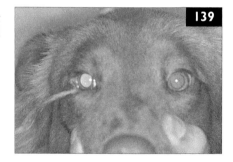

140 A 10-year-old female German Shepherd Dog presents for annual vaccinations. On ocular examination the nucleus of the lens has increased opacification and there are large multiple punctate opacities in both eyes (140a).
i. What is the diagnosis?
ii. What is the pathophysiology of this condition?
iii. What is the treatment?

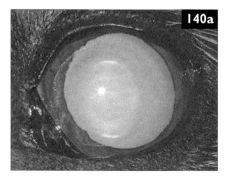

138 i. The kitten has a large iris prolapse and a corneal abscess.
ii. The kitten was so eager to eat that she managed to cover her face in food!
iii. The globe was gently enucleated and the kitten recovered nicely.

139 i. An eyelid dermoid. Dermoids of the lids are ectopic islands of skin in or at the margin of the eyelid. They are frequently associated with some dysplastic deformities of the adjacent conjunctiva. They are usually found on the lower lid near the lateral canthus. Genetic predisposition exists in the German Shepherd Dog, Dalmatian, and St. Bernard. Blinking is abnormal and hairs generally grow towards the cornea, causing chronic irritation and resulting in edema, vascularization, and pigmentation.
ii. Treatment consists of removal of the abnormal parts of the eyelid and conjunctiva, and especially the malpositioned hair follicles in the involved area. Blepharoplasties are necessary when lid margin involvement is extensive.

140 i. Nuclear sclerosis and a nuclear cataract.
ii. Fully developed normal lens fibers consist of long, rod-shaped cells with distinct 'ball and socket' intercellular attachments that allow the lens fibers to change shape during accommodation. In cataracts, these lens cells swell (**140b**, scanning electron micrograph of a swollen lens fiber) as cell membrane integrity is reduced. As a result, the structural uniformity of the fibers where the swelling occurs is lost, and the ability of light to transmit through this region is impeded. It often begins with small opacities that eventually coalesce, block light, and affect vision. Nuclear sclerosis is an age-related opacification of the lens associated with nuclear dehydration and altered lens proteins. It is not a true cataract.
iii. Lens removal is warranted if vision loss is severe, but was not performed in this dog as she had functional vision.

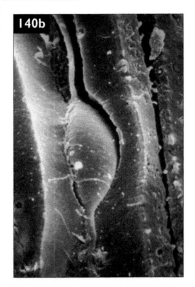

140b

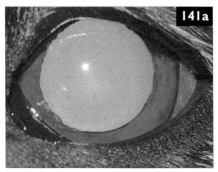

141 For comparison with the 10-year-old female German Shepherd Dog in case 140, an 11-year-old female Labrador Retriever is examined for blue eyes. Retroillumination through a dilated pupil shows a central dense nucleus with a surrounding clear halo (141a).
i. What is the diagnosis?
ii. What is the pathophysiology of this condition?
iii. What is the treatment?

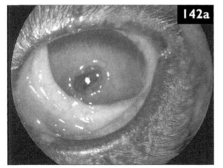
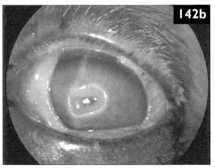

142 In this patient an acute corneal ulcer has formed (142a) due to a sudden onset of keratoconjunctivitis sicca (KCS) caused by administration of a systemic antibiotic. Note how fluorescein does not stain the center of the ulcer (142b).
i. Describe the clinical signs in the two photographs?
ii. What is the diagnosis of this corneal problem?
iii. What is the proposed mechanism of KCS caused by sulfa antibiotics?
iv. What are the immediate concerns associated with the corneal problem?
v. What diagnostic test should always be performed on this corneal problem prior to surgical repair?
vi. How should this case be managed surgically?

141 i. Nuclear sclerosis.
ii. The pathophysiology is a dense nucleus, which is not a true pathologic process. As the lens ages, it compresses the lens fibers (**141b,** scanning electron micrograph of older lens fibers that have become more accordion in shape, but concomitantly have lost their flexibility) in the nucleus to make room for new lens fibers. The nucleus becomes relatively dehydrated and compacted such that it is no longer perfectly transparent. The lens fiber arrangement is still relatively normal. The older the animal, the more dense the nucleus.
iii. There is no treatment. As long as the center of the lens is transparent the animal should be visual, though the ability to fine tune vision via lenticular accommodation becomes increasingly

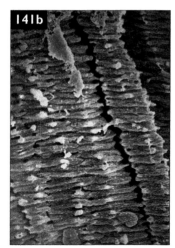

diminished with age until it is entirely lost. This effect is believed to have minimal influence on the visual behavior of small domestic animals.

142 i. There is protrusion of a moderately hyperemic and chemotic nictitating membrane, moderate diffuse corneal edema, and a deep black depression or descemetocele of the axial cornea. The depression edges are fluorescein positive and the depression center is fluorescein negative.
ii. A descemetocele, which results from exposure of Descemet's membrane. Descemet's membrane does not stain with fluorescein (see case **194**) and it is only about 3–12 μm thick in dogs. Corneal ulcers that are deep enough to become descemetoceles can be due to infection, excessive tear film protease activity, or traumatic injury. In this case the deep corneal ulcer has been caused by KCS secondary to the use of oral sulfonamide antibiotics.
iii. A toxic effect of the drug on the lacrimal glands. In some cases, lacrimation returns to normal after cessation of administration of the antibiotic if the antibiotic was only used for a short term. Long-term use may lead to a permanent dry eye condition.
iv. Due to the thin nature of a descemetocele, rupture of the globe is imminent.
v. Bacterial and fungal culture should be performed on all descemetoceles prior to surgical repair.
vi. Conjunctival flaps or amnion grafts should be considered. A conjunctival flap can provide structural support as well as a direct blood supply to the affected area. If available, corneal grafting or a corneoscleral transposition are also acceptable surgical options.

143 This dog was presented with a melting corneal ulcer and corneal cellular infiltrate (143a). The ulcer was swabbed for culture. Culture of the cornea revealed infection with *Pseudomonas* spp.
i. What is the pathophysiology of the melting ulcer in this dog?
ii. What is the benefit of a pedicle conjunctival flap?

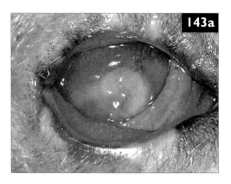

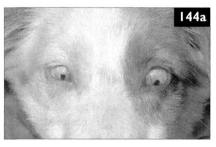

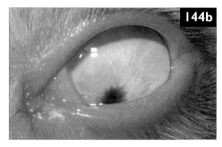

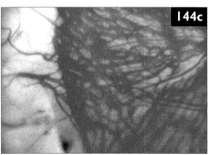

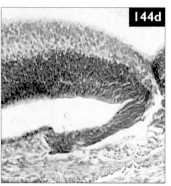

144 An Australian Shepherd Dog puppy is presented with these multiple congenital ocular defects (144a–d). Microphthalmos is present in both eyes. The pupils are dyscoric. Fundus examination reveals an equatorial coloboma with a retinal tear.
i. What is a coloboma, and how does it form embryologically?
ii. What is the syndrome called that is associated with equatorial colobomas in the Australian Shepherd Dog?
iii. Describe the histologic appearance of the equatorial coloboma in Australian Shepherd Dogs.

143 i. Opportunistic infections by bacteria are common in corneal ulcers. Many cases of melting ulcers in dogs and cats involve *Pseudomonas* spp. Such ulcers are often rapidly progressing melting ulcers that require prompt surgical therapy. Culture and sensitivity of the ulcer should be performed prior to surgery, and the initial antimicrobial therapy adjusted based on the results. For more details about the patho-physiology and treatment of melting ulcers, see case **137**.

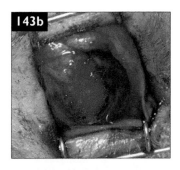

ii. The use of pedicle conjunctival flaps (**143b, c**) covering only a small area of the normal cornea allows the clinician to visualize much of the cornea and anterior chamber, which in turn allows continuous examination of these structures in order to monitor ulcer progression and possible anterior uveitis. Having only a small portion of the cornea covered may also allow the animal to continue to be visual. Hood conjunctival flaps or

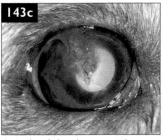

nictitans flaps will cause blindness in the eye for the length of the therapy. Three to eight weeks after placement of the grafts, the blood supply should be interrupted by cutting the base of the graft at the limbus. This can usually be performed using topical anesthesia and Stevens tenotomy scissors. Eliminating the blood supply will allow the conjunctival graft to recede and lessen the resulting corneal scar.

144 i. A coloboma is a tissue defect (**144c**, funduscopic view of a coloboma). Embryologically, colobomas in Australian Shepherd Dogs form due to a primary defect and reduced formation of the retinal pigmented epithelium (RPE), which in turn results in focal hypoplasia of the choroid and sclera (see case **87**).

ii. Merle ocular dysgenesis, a syndrome accompanied by microphthalmia, microcornea, heterochromia irides, dyscoria, corectopia, iris hypoplasia, cataracts, retinal detachment, and scleral colobomas.

iii. The coloboma, when examined histopathologically, shows decreased to absent choroidal vasculature in the location concomitant with an absent RPE, and a thin and irregular sclera that seals off the defect. The retina cannot attach to an RPE-less area and has the potential of becoming dysplastic. In **144d** (light microscopic view) the retina is seen to come together where the choroidal fissure failed to close properly and the RPE had ceased to form.

145 A nine-month-old Shih Tzu is presented with a two-week history of blepharospasm, epiphora, corneal edema, and corneal vascularization. Fluorescein has been applied topically (145a).
i. What is your diagnosis?
ii. What is a likely cause for this condition in a young brachycephalic dog?
iii. What are the treatment options?

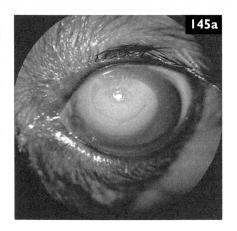

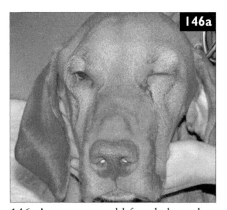

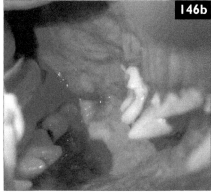

146 A seven-year-old female hound was presented at the clinic with an inflamed left orbit (146a). The owner noted that the dog had lost her appetite over the past couple of days and that a discharged substance was draining down the left side of her face. The dog was quite sensitive to slight pressure applied around the left orbit as well as when looking into her mouth. There was no doubt that she was in considerable pain. The discharge was mostly mucopurulent in content. There was swelling of the oral mucosa, primarily behind the last ipsilateral molar (146b). Blood count analysis revealed a high neutrophil count (neutrophilia).
i. What is the most likely diagnosis? Do you expect the eye to be involved directly?
ii. What is the recommended therapy?

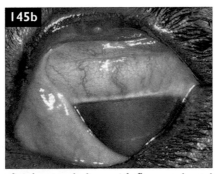

145 i. There is a superficial corneal ulcer, with fluorescein staining under the visible edge of the ulcer. This is an indolent ulcer. The stain has diffused under the loose edge of the ulcer, creating a larger area of fluorescein uptake than the exposed stroma.

ii. Indolent corneal ulcers in brachycephalic dogs can be primary or secondary to eyelash or eyelid abnormalities, corneal edema, infection, or tear film abnormalities. Ectopic cilia grow down from the meibomian gland and exit through the palpebral conjunctiva, as in this case (145b). This nearly always occurs near the center of the upper lid. The hairs can often be very small and require magnification to be observed. Fluorescein stain may coat the ectopic cilia and make them easier to visualize. Animals with ectopic cilia often have severe ocular pain and chronic corneal ulcers. Diagnosis is made with the eyelid everted to look for a papilla of tissue containing the hair(s).

iii. Conjunctival resection is the preferred treatment.

146 i. This dog most likely has an orbital or retrobulbar abscess or cellulitis. The eye is expected to be uninvolved in most of these cases.

ii. In this instance the eye appeared normal and the intraocular pressure was normal. Administration of systemic antibiotics is strongly indicated. There is rarely a discrete abscess to drain, but careful surgical drainage of an orbital abscess or pocket of cellulitis is very important in cases that recur following administration of antibiotics.

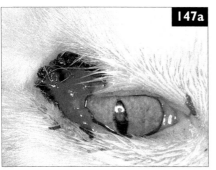 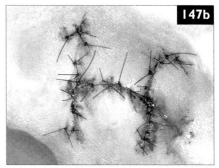

147 You are presented with an older white-haired domestic shorthaired cat with an ulcerated lesion on the right dorsolateral eyelid (147a). There is no history of trauma and the owner indicates that the cat lives indoors.
i. Based on the presentation, what is the likely diagnosis?
ii. Discuss the etiology and pathophysiology of this lesion.
iii. What surgery is being performed in 147b.

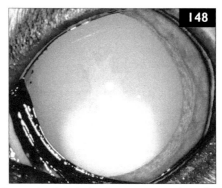

148 A 10-year-old domestic shorthaired cat presents for what the owner describes as 'the sudden development of a cataract' (148).
i. Discuss the formation of a cataract in the cat.
ii. Would you recommend surgery to remove the cataract?

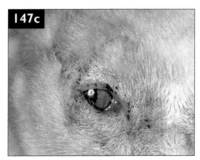

147 i. A squamous cell carcinoma (SCC).
ii. SCCs are the most common tumors of the eyelids in cats. Their prevalence increases with age and they are most common in white cats. These tumors are usually associated with the eyelid margin, are ulcerated or crusted, and are slightly raised. Although metastasis is only likely if the disease is allowed to progress, the tumor can be locally very aggressive.
iii. While cryotherapy and teletherapy/radiation therapy are often effective against SCCs, the most effective treatment is surgical removal. An H-flap technique (H-type blepharoplasty) was used to excise the tumor in this cat. An H-flap is effective for the excision of full-thickness eyelid neoplasms. This is a sliding skin graft that uses a graft of skin distal to the neoplasm. Initially, two incisions are made to either side of the tumor. Then two equal-sized triangles are cut at the extent of the linear incisions. The tumor is removed, followed by careful dissection of the graft and suturing of the graft over the defect left by the tumor. This is a relatively simple procedure that is effective and leaves very little lid scarring (**147c**, two months postoperatively the incisions have healed).

148 i. Primary and inherited cataracts are not as common in cats as they are in dogs. The majority of cataracts in the cat are secondary to trauma, uveitis, diabetes, lens luxation, or glaucoma. This is a Morgagnian-type cataract. The more opaque and heavy lens nucleus has settled out ventrally because of gravity when the cataract in the outer cortex resorbs and liquefies. Uveitis is often associated with Morgagnian cataracts, which are considered a variant of the hypermature cataract. The lens capsule is wrinkled in these cataracts due to cortex resorption.
ii. Phacoemulsification is performed in cats and is reported to have a greater success rate than in dogs. The uvea of cats is less reactive to the trauma of surgery and postoperative inflammation more readily controlled, resulting in a high success rate.

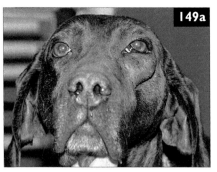
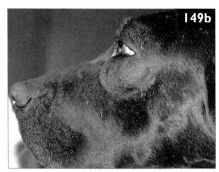

149 This middle-aged Labrador Retriever has developed a soft swelling below the left eye (149a, b).
i. What are the differentials for such a lesion?
ii. What diagnostic tests and therapy are indicated?

150 A three-year-old Siamese cat was presented with a brown colored mass visible in the right eye (150).
i. Describe the lesion.
ii. What are the two major differentials?
iii. What is the pathophysiology of this condition?
iv. What are the treatment options?

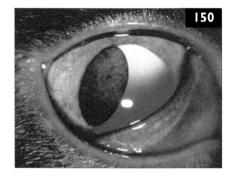

151 A six-year-old Pekingese was presented one week ago for proptosis (151). The proptosis was repaired, but the owner is worried because the dog 'doesn't move his eye correctly any-more'.
i. What has occurred in this case?
ii. What caused this condition for this particular dog?
iii. Can this condition be treated?

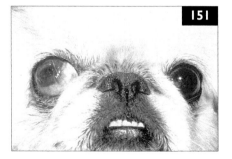

149 i. Zygomatic salivary gland adenitis, sialocele, or neoplasia; zygomatic bone neoplasia; dental problems.
ii. Fine-needle aspirate and/or biopsy, oral and orbital examination, and imaging with CT/MRI and plain films could aid the diagnosis. The fine-needle aspirate indicated a zygomatic salivary gland adenitis that responded to systemic antibiotics.

150 i. There is a brown oval-shaped mass in the lateral pupil margin. The mass appears to be behind the iris and is comparable to that seen in case 27.
ii. Uveal melanoma and an iridal cyst. The easiest way to differentiate between these two is to transilluminate the mass (see cases 27 and 53). An iridal cyst will allow light from the tapetal reflection to show back through the mass (see the dorsal part of the mass in 150). Melanomas will not transilluminate because they are solid tissue. Ocular ultrasound can be performed to help diagnose masses that are difficult to transilluminate.
iii. The pathophysiology of iridal cysts is localized dilation of the margin of the optic vesicle after it forms the optic cup. Cysts can be single or multiple and can be free floating or attached to the posterior iris or the pupillary margin.
iv. Iridal cysts are not treated unless the mass is impairing vision. Cysts that are impairing vision, obstructing aqueous flow, or causing mechanical damage to the corneal endothelium can be treated with laser deflation.

151 i. This dog has strabismus secondary to the globe proptosis. Strabismus is a common complication of traumatic globe proptosis.
ii. Extraocular muscles are commonly torn or avulsed secondary to globe proptosis. The most susceptible muscles are the medial and ventral rectus muscles and the ventral oblique muscle. When only one muscle has been torn, the strabismus may be a temporary complication. If three or more extraocular muscles are torn, the prognosis is less favorable. In this particular dog the ventral rectus and ventral oblique were likely ruptured, resulting in a dorsolateral strabismus.
iii. If necessary, the positioning of the extraocular muscles can be repaired. However, if only a partial tear has occurred, the deviations can spontaneously decrease within a few months. Any exposed bulbar conjunctiva will become pigmented and diminish the awkward appearance in time.

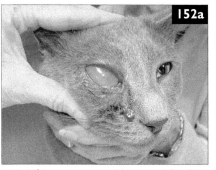
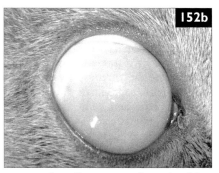

152 This cat returned home with what the owner describes as an enlarged, white-blue eye (152a, b). The cat is painful, exhibits epiphora and blepharospasm, and is vocalizing. The cornea is fluorescein negative. There are no right direct or left consensual pupillary light reflexes.
i. What is the most likely diagnosis?
ii. What is the pathophysiology of this disease?
iii. What other diagnostic tests might aid the diagnosis?
iv. How would you treat this cat?

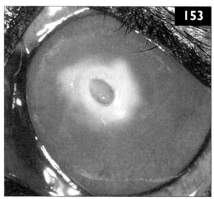

153 A three-year-old mixed breed dog was presented with an axial iris prolapse. The coloring seen (153) is the result of topically administered fluorescein.
i. Describe the ocular findings.
ii. What is the treatment for this problem?

152 i. Endophthalmitis, most likely caused by a foreign body or penetrating wound to the eye.

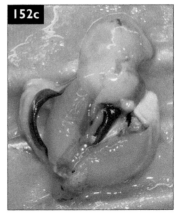

ii. Endophthalmitis occurs following penetration of the eye by a foreign body or claw that can impregnate the vitreous, anterior chamber, and cornea with bacteria. It can also occur from endogenous systemic infections. Bacterial infection leads to inflammation, neutrophil migration, and purulent exudate formation. Corneal edema results from severe uveitis. The intraocular pressure was elevated due to angle obstruction with inflammatory debris.

iii. This eye is enlarged (buphthalmic), has severe corneal edema, and contains a large amount of purulent material in the anterior chamber. Ultrasound would be an excellent additional diagnostic tool to assess the intraocular environment and ocular structure. Endophthalmitis will result in the presence of hyperechoic debris in the anterior chambers and vitreous. Tonometry is important to check intraocular pressure.

iv. The most humane course of treatment in this case is enucleation. The pus-filled globe following enucleation in this cat is shown (152c).

153 i. There is moderate, diffuse corneal edema with an axial superficial ulcer (with fluorescein uptake). At the center of the superficial ulcer is a corneal perforation with iris prolapse covered in reddish fibrin.

ii. Full-thickness corneal perforations can develop from the progression of deep corneal ulcers or from trauma. The iris moves anteriorly to plug the hole in the cornea. Because of the risk for infection and intraocular inflammatory damage with perforations, surgical repair of the lesions should be recommended. Before surgery, the potential for vision of the affected eye should be assessed. Evaluation of the consensual pupillary light and dazzle reflexes may provide some information regarding the integrity of the retina and posterior segment. Corneal perforations should be considered at risk of infection, and preoperative bacterial culture and sensitivity tests performed before surgery to help direct medical therapy. Corneal perforations have been treated successfully with conjunctival grafts, amnion transplants, and corneal transplants. Bioengineered porcine small intestinal submucosa and extracellular matrix derived from porcine urinary bladder have been used for the replacement of missing cornea.

154 This one-year-old mixed breed dog was presented with blepharospasm of both eyes (154).
i. What are the possible reasons for blepharospasm?
ii. How should you determine the cause?

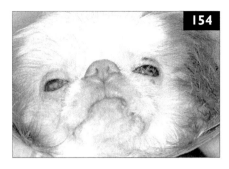

155 You are presented with a cat who is exhibiting generalized depression, fever, inappetence, and weight loss. On examination you also note corneal abnormalities consistent with 'mutton-fat' keratitic precipitates (KPs) and hyphema (155).
i. What disease is this cat suffering from?
ii. Describe the disease and the pathophysiology of the ocular changes.
iii. What is the prognosis for this cat?

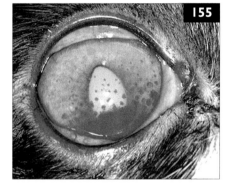

156 A dog has a melting ulcer. When fluorescein dye is placed on the cornea and not flushed off, a progressive change in fluorescein color is noted to occur (156). What is the problem here?

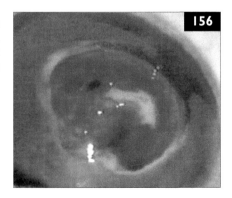

154 i. Blepharospasm is spasm of the eyelid muscle resulting in closure of the eyelids. It is caused by conjunctival, corneal, and/or intraocular pain, or by stimulation of the palpebral nerve. Painful ocular conditions can be caused by corneal ulcers, glaucoma, uveitis, keratoconjunctivitis sicca, foreign bodies, and by distichia, trichiasis, and ectopic cilia. Ocular pain may cause the globe to be retracted into the orbit and result in secondary third eyelid elevation.
ii. Thorough eye examination, including biomicroscopy, tonometry, and a Schirmer tear test (STT), should reveal the source of pain leading to the blepharospasm. In this case the intraocular pressure was within normal limits and no foreign body or lid hair disorders were found. STT was 5 mm/60 seconds and biomicroscopy revealed superficial keratitis and conjunctivitis. Blepharospasm, accompanied by enophthalmos in this case, resulted from the pain and discomfort caused by deficiency of the precorneal tear film.

155 i. Feline infectious peritonitis (FIP).
ii. FIP is a coronavirus that can present in two different forms, effusive and non-effusive (see cases 177 and 229). Vasculitis causes the clinical signs of effusive FIP. The granulatomous nature of the disease leads to the deposition of 'mutton-fat' KPs on the cornea, as seen in 155. Pyogranulomatous chorioretinitis and perivascular cuffing can also result.
iii. Currently, there is no treatment for this disease. A definitive diagnosis is made at necropsy. Palliative care with corticosteroid therapy and symptomatic treatment is the only treatment option.

156 This is a positive Seidel's test and it indicates a hole in the cornea, with leakage of aqueous humor through the hole. The orange fluorescein dye color is altered to become green or clear when aqueous humor leaks through the corneal hole and dilutes the fluorescein. A Seidel's test should be utilized in all deep ulcers and following suture placement in a cornea.

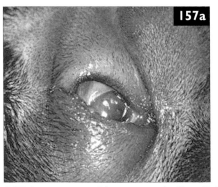
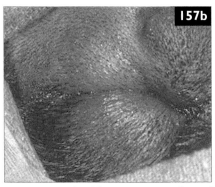

157 A two-year-old intact male Shar Pei was presented with severe entropion of both eyes (157a, b). Describe the surgical technique used to correct both the entropion and the trichiasis in one procedure.

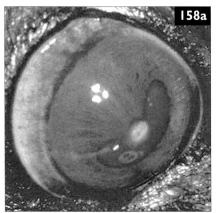
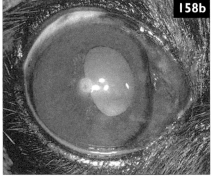

158 A one-year-old mixed breed rescue dog is presented for ocular examination. A small lesion is detected near the center of the cornea (158a, b).
i. Describe the lesion.
ii. What is the most likely diagnosis?
iii. What is the most common etiology?
iv. What are the potential long-term complications?

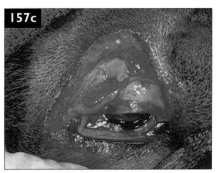

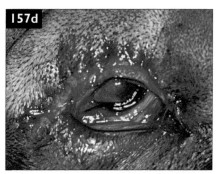

157 The Stades procedure combines correction of upper eyelid trichiasis and entropion (157c, d). A section of upper eyelid skin is excised extending vertically 0.5–1.0 mm from the upper lid margin to 15–25 mm above the palpebral fissure, and horizontally 2–4 mm medial from the nasal canthus to 5–10 mm external to the lateral canthus. The upper eyelid wound is partially closed by apposition of the upper eyelid skin to the subcutaneous eyelid layer 5–6 mm from the eyelid margin with 4-0 to 5-0 simple interrupted sutures or a combination of simple interrupted and continuous nonabsorbable suture. The exposed area immediately above the upper eyelid margin heals by secondary intention and the resultant fibrosis everts the upper eyelid margin. This area may become pigmented. The animal still retains its facial folds of skin and its overall appearance is not markedly altered in the Stades procedure.

158 i. There is a small oval-shaped opacity in the cornea. In the center of the opacity there is a brown pigmented area. The pupil is dyscoric (abnormal shape) and the iris on the left is pulled up toward the cornea.
ii. A healed corneal perforation, small iris prolapse, and an anterior synechia.
iii. Trauma, such as a cat scratch, or puncture from a foreign body.
iv. The perforated cornea can heal with an anterior synechia if the perforation is very small, as in this dog. Complications can include intraocular infection and associated lens trauma. The inciting injury can damage the cornea and lens capsule such that it may cause uveitis and cataract formation (see cases 35 and 153).

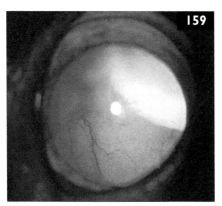

159 A 13-year-old Tonkinese cat presents with acute bilateral blindness.
i. Describe the lesion seen in 159.
ii. What is the diagnosis?
iii. What are the differentials for this condition?
iv. What test should be performed?
v. What is the pathophysiology of this condition?

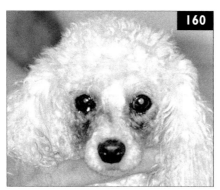

160 This eight-month-old Toy Poodle was brought into the clinic with obvious discoloration below each eye (160).
i. Describe the clinical findings.
ii. Explain the pathophysiology of this condition and possible treatment.

159 i. There is a membrane of tissue with vessels just posterior to the lens.
ii. Bullous retinal detachment.
iii. The main differential for a bullous retinal detachment in a 13-year-old cat is systemic hypertension, until proven otherwise.
iv. Any cat presenting for acute bilateral blindness should have its blood pressure evaluated. Cats with hypertensive retinopathy often have systolic blood pressures 160–200 mmHg or greater.
v. The eye is the target organ for hypertensive damage. The small diameter vessels in the eye vasoconstrict when there is prolonged systemic hypertension. The vasoconstriction is normally autoregulated, but this autoregulation breaks down under conditions of high blood pressure, resulting in compromised vascular integrity. Leakage of plasma and red blood cells occurs when the endothelial cells and vascular smooth muscle become damaged. This leakage leads to retinal edema and focal fluid accumulation within the neurosensory layer. Retinal detachment is the result of this effusion from the diseased choroidal vasculature.

160 i. Bilateral epiphora with nasal tear staining.
ii. Many brachycephalic and toy breed dogs have epiphora and tear staining related to a reduced rate of tear drainage rather than excessive tear production due to multiple anomalies of the medial canthal region and inferior puncta. The inferior puncta and canaliculi are commonly displaced inward and ventrally by a subtle, nasoventral entropion, which rolls the medial eyelid margin into the cornea, partially obstructs the puncta, and narrows and compresses the canalicular lumen. In addition, tight medial canthal ligaments displace the medial canthus ventrally and, in combination with medial canthal trichiasis and eyelid trichiasis, exacerbate tear spillage in these dogs. The brown color results from bacterial action on the tear film proteins.

The treatment of choice for this condition is observation and daily cleaning with dermatologic ointments and hydrogen peroxide, or a bilateral medial canthoplasty to correct the caruncular trichiasis and tighten medial canthal ligaments. Systemic antibiotics can reduce the tear staining in severe cases.

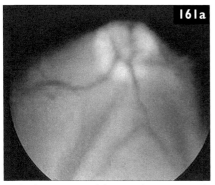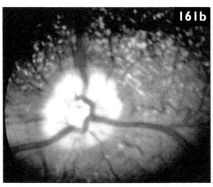

161 A six-year-old spayed German Shepherd Dog was presented for ophthalmic examination with a complaint of blindness. Fundic pictures were taken before treatment (161a) and 30 days post treatment (161b).
i. What is the diagnosis, and give an explanation of the cause of the pathology shown in 161a?
ii. What is the etiology of the problem in this dog?
iii. How would you treat the dog?

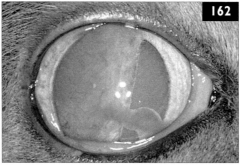

162 A cat was presented with a large growth over 75% of the iris that was obliterating the anterior chamber (162). The owner reported that the growth had been present for several months, but had recently significantly increased in size.
i. What are the differential diagnoses?
ii. What are the treatment options?
iii. What is the prognosis for this cat?

161 **i.** Exudative, bullous retinal detachment. Retinal detachment is actually the separation of the retina between the photoreceptor layers and the pigment epithelium. The intimate contact between the rods and cones and pigment epithelial cells is disrupted, leading to retinal hypoxia. The normal pumping mechanism to remove subretinal waste products and fluid no longer functions, such that fluid accumulates in the subretinal space to form large bullae and push the retina anteriorly. Fluid and cell deposition in the subretinal space can occur from chorioretinitis or vascular hypertension. Large volumes of subretinal fluid can cause the retina to balloon anteriorly, even extending to the posterior surface of the lens in extreme cases. When there is anterior displacement of the detached retina it can often be readily viewed directly through the pupil with a focal light source.
ii. Exudative retinal detachment, for which an etiology is not established despite laboratory work-up, has been recognized for many years in large breed dogs and termed steroid-responsive retinal detachment. Affected dogs typically present with a history of an acute-onset loss of vision. The detachments are bilateral and nonrhegmatogenous (no holes in the retina). German Shepherd Dogs and Labrador crosses are commonly affected.
iii. Even extensive detachments may be reattached, with return of vision provided treatment is commenced early (**161b**). When a steroid-responsive exudative detachment is suspected, systemic steroids should be started as soon as possible after ruling out potential infectious and systemic causes. Failure to reattach leads to retinal degeneration and loss of visual capacity in the affected area.

162 **i.** Differentials include lymphoma, melanoma, and adenoma. Melanomas are the most common primary intraocular tumor in the cat and, as in the dog, they can be amelanotic in nature.
ii. Uveal melanomas in cats can be either relatively benign if nodular, or malignant if they are diffuse in nature. Treatment is by enucleation.
iii. The prognosis for life is generally good. Melanomas are generally not as highly aggressive as other ocular tumors. Nevertheless, metastasis can occur and enucleation is recommended (see case **118**).

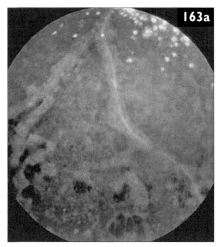

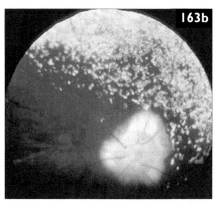

163 A seven-year-old Miniature Poodle is presented with depression and sudden loss of vision. The owner complains that the dog has been bumping into walls in the last couple of days. These images are obtained from direct ophthalmoscopy (163a, b).
i. Describe what you see in these fundic images.
ii. What are the possible causes of the vision loss in this dog?
iii. What is the most likely diagnosis?
iv. What is the pathophysiology of this disease?

164 A six-month-old kitten is presented with an acute, gray, soft spot in the cornea (164).
i. What are the differentials for this condition?
ii. What is the most likely diagnosis?
iii. What diagnostic tests should be performed?
iv. What is the etiology of this condition?
v. What are the treatment options?

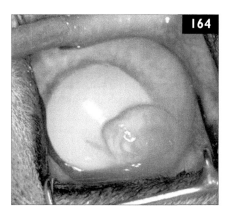

163 i. Attenuation of the retinal vasculature and the presence of 'ghost vessels', which have developed in response to retinal atrophy. The optic disk is visible in 163b and appears normal in color and shape. The periphery of the nontapetum has a grayish discoloration and there is mild tapetal hyperreflectivity (163a).
ii. The retinal disease could be the result of drug toxicity, vitamin E deficiency, or progressive retinal atrophy (PRA). Optic neuritis and sudden acquired retinal degeneration could also be causes of this appearance.
iii. Considering the signalment in this case, PRA or, more specifically, progressive rod-cone degeneration (Prcd) is the most likely diagnosis.
iv. Prcd is an autosomal recessive trait common to many breeds of dog, including the Miniature and Toy Poodle, Cocker Spaniel, Labrador Retriever, Portuguese Water Dog, and Australian Cattle Dog. The prevalence in Poodles is particularly high. The disease manifests as early as three years of age and usually begins with the development of night blindness. Pathology actually begins to develop in puppies as early as 12–14 weeks of age. The degenerative process begins in the inferior retinal quadrants and progresses to the superior and temporal quadrants later in the disease. The rod physiology is affected before the cones develop pathology, but both photoreceptors are eventually damaged.

164 i. Differentials include bullous keratopathy, descemetocele, corneal foreign body, iris prolapse, melting corneal ulcer, epithelial inclusion cyst, and corneal endothelial dystrophy.
ii. Bullous keratopathy. This acute condition often presents bilaterally in cats and may lead to corneal perforation (for a different example see case 99).
iii. A Seidel's test should be performed to help determine if there is aqueous humor leaking through a corneal perforation. Corneal cytology and culture should be obtained.
iv. There are several theories for feline bullous keratopathy. Endothelial dystrophy, as in the Manx cat, excessive stromal protease activity, and uveitis disrupting corneal endothelial function can result in bulla formation. The condition is often linked to previous use of topical steroids.
v. Aggressive medical therapy and surgery. Medical therapy for this condition includes topical anti-collagenases (EDTA, serum, N-acetylcysteine), broad-spectrum antibiotics, mydriatics, and hypertonic saline (5% NaCl). Surgical options, if the eye is not ruptured, include a nictitans flap and/or a tarsorrhaphy.

165 A 14-year-old mixed breed dog is presented with unilateral lower eyelid (left) swelling and mild mucoid discharge (165a).
i. The basic ophthalmic examination was normal. What other test can be performed to determine if there is a bulbar mass?
ii. What is the next step?
iii. What is the treatment?

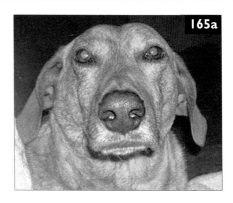

166 This cat (166) has a dilated pupil and a negative dazzle reflex. What is present in this eye?

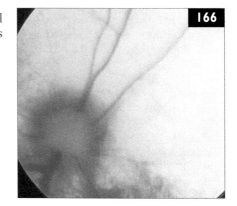

167 A six–week-old kitten is presented with symblepharon (167).
i. What is the leading cause of symblepharon in cats?
ii. What are the treatment options?

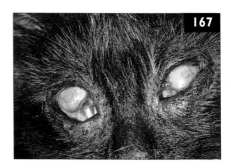

165 i. Retropulsion of the globe. The lids are gently closed manually over the globes and both eyes are simultaneously pushed gently back into the orbits. The affected eye will not retropulse are well as the normal eye if there is an orbital mass. Pain may be elicited in some cases. The retropulsion was normal and without pain in this dog.
ii. An oral examination. In older dogs, a thorough dental examination of the upper molars on the affected side is indicated. A tooth root abscess (165b) was found to be responsible for causing the swelling in this dog and in case 146.

iii. Extraction of the affected tooth to treat the tooth abscess and digital radiography post extraction to evaluate residual root apices. The tooth sockets should be gently curetted to open any abscess pockets. Broad-spectrum antibiotics should be started pending culture results. The lower lid swelling and ocular discharge should completely resolve in 7–10 days.

166 The normally sharp and distinct outline of the optic disk of this cat is fuzzy and out of focus. The diagnosis is optic neuritis. Optic neuritis is rare in cats and is associated with feline infectious peritonitis, toxoplasmosis, and cryptococcosis.

167 i. Herpesvirus conjunctivitis. In some cats, conjunctivitis can become severe, with the result that ulcerations of the conjunctival epithelium occur. Ulcerated areas in the conjunctiva can form adhesions to one another and to ulcerated corneal lesions. These adhered areas can become permanent (symblepharon) if not broken down quickly. Symblepharon can involve the entire corneal ocular surface.
ii. A conjunctival transposition of resecting, moving the symblepharon adhesion back to the conjunctiva, and then suturing it to the sclera has been reported. Covering the remaining corneal ulcer with amnion can also prevent recurrence. Topical cyclosporin A and flurbiprofen may also help by reducing the inflammation during healing.

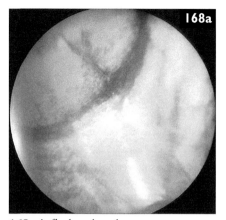

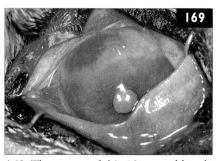

169 The owner of this 13-year-old male Basset Hound was concerned with what she saw and brought her dog with the presenting ophthalmic problem (**169**).
i. Describe the clinical findings.
ii. What are the differential diagnoses?
iii. What is the treatment?

168 A flesh-colored mass was present in the vitreous and retina of this domestic shorthaired adult cat (**168a**). What is the differential diagnosis for this condition?

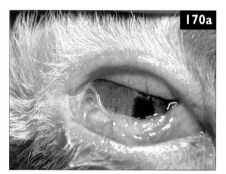

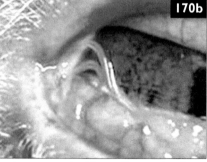

170 A four-year-old domestic shorthaired cat is presented with swelling and redness of the eyes. The owner says the cat has been slightly uncomfortable for two weeks, but it seems to be getting worse. She explains that the cat lives in the barn with the horses and cows and is usually quite independent, but lately has been staying around the barn more. The ophthalmic examination reveals small white motile strands within the conjunctiva and on the cornea (**170a, b**).
i. What are these small, white strands?
ii. Describe how this infection occurs.
iii. What is the treatment?

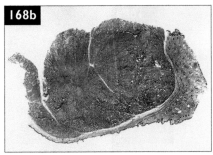

168 This is a cat with a ciliary body tumor that is causing retinal degeneration and retinal detachment. Uveal neoplasia in the cat is most commonly due to lympho-sarcoma, plasma cell myeloma, carcinoma, or adenocarcinoma. The tumor in this cat was determined to be an adenoma (168b, light microscopy of uveal adenoma), which occupied space normally occupied by the vitreous.

169 i. A dorsally-located (between nine and two o'clock) fleshy corneal mass, bordered by corneal edema and vascularization, occupies about 25% of the cornea.
ii. Include squamous cell carcinoma, lymphosarcoma, hemangioma, hemangio-sarcoma, and adenocarcinoma. In young dogs, viral papillomas should also considered. Diagnosis is determined by biopsy. In this case the diagnosis was hemangiosarcoma of the cornea, which is uncommon in the dog, but is fairly destructive when it arises. Hemangiosarcomas are commonly accompanied by extensive corneal vascularization and perilesional edema.
iii. Therapy includes corneoscleral graft or enucleation.

170 i. The nematode *Thelazia californiensis*. This worm can be found within the conjunctival sac under the third eyelid and in the lacrimal duct.
ii. Infection with *Thelazia* spp. begins with ingestion of the larvae from the tears by flies. The larvae develop in the fly for about 30 days and are then redeposited on the eye of a host when the fly feeds near the eye. The larvae grow into adults, which are approximately 10–14 mm long. The adults feed off the secretions of the eye. Damage to the conjunctiva results from the lateral serration of the cuticle of the larvae.
iii. Treatment consists of physical removal of the parasites. Topical parasiticides could be useful in selected cases.

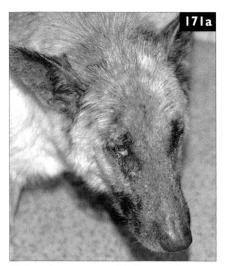

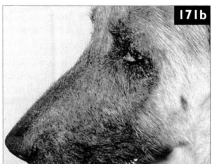

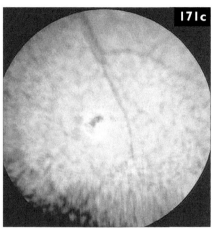

171 A ten-year-old intact German Shepherd Dog survived canine distemper virus (CDV) infection. He now suffers from demodicosis associated with chronic infection with CDV as well as the ocular complications shown (171a–c). What are the possible ocular complications of CDV infection?

172 Transcleral cyclophotocoagulation in a dog is shown (172).
i. What is this technique utilized for?
ii. What is the mode of action of this therapy?

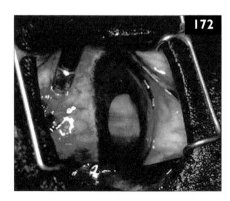

171 Bilateral mucoid conjunctivitis is an early sign of CDV infection that appears within the first week of exposure to the virus. With time the discharge becomes mucopurulent and the cytologic response changes from mononuclear to polymorphonuclear. Cytoplasmic inclusion bodies are uncommon, but can be present in conjunctival epithelial cells early in the infection (**171d**, distemper inclusion (1) from conjunctival cytology). CDV causes adenitis of the

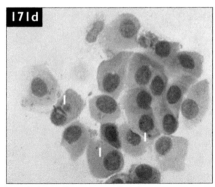

lacrimal glands and the glands of the third eyelid, and may result in a transient or permanent keratoconjunctivitis sicca. Acute solitary or multifocal chorioretinitis occurs frequently in dogs with CDV infection. The appearance of retinal lesions (**171c**, 'medallion' lesion) is similar to that of retinitis from other causes, with areas of retinal atrophy manifested by tapetal hyperreflectivity and pigmentation. The effect on vision is variable depending on the distribution and number of retinal lesions. Optic neuritis is associated with CDV. Central blindness may develop as a consequence of chronic distemper-induced encephalitis, which results in demyelination and astrocytosis of the optic radiations.

172 **i.** The treatment of glaucoma.
ii. Transcleral cyclophotocoagulation decreases the formation rate of aqueous humor by destroying part of the ciliary body. Laser energy directed through the overlying sclera results in high heat and coagulation of the epithelium of the pigmented ciliary body processes. In the dog the probe must be positioned approximately 5 mm posterior to the limbus in order to reach the ciliary body processes. With globe enlargement, the ciliary processes of the pars plicata may shift an additional 0.5–1.0 mm posteriorly. Moderate laser energy levels can be used to lower intraocular pressure in visual eyes, but excessive application of laser energy can result in irreversible destruction of the ciliary body, permanent ocular hypotony, and phthisis bulbi. In nonpigmented eyes (e.g. as in the Siberian Husky), laser cyclophotocoagulation is less successful.

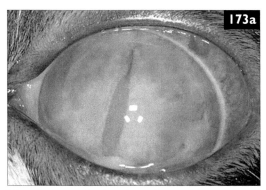

173 A 13-year-old male domestic shorthaired cat with a two-month history of iris color change and a two-week history of ocular pain is examined (173a).
i. Describe the lesion.
ii. What are the differentials?
iii. What is the treatment?

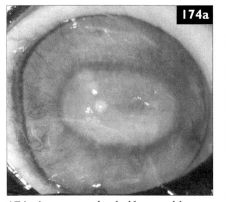

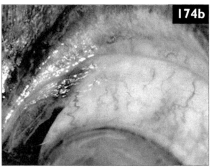

174 A seven-and-a-half-year-old neutered Belgian Shepherd Dog was presented with an axial ulcer and corneal edema. The ulcer was treated with no effect with triple antibiotic eye ointment three times a day. After 14 days of therapy the dog was referred to a veterinary ophthalmologist. The eye examination revealed extensive corneal changes.
i. Describe the clinical findings shown (174a, b).
ii. What are the possible causes for this?

173 i. There is moderate bulbar con-junctival hyperemia, a superficial fluorescein-positive corneal ulcer, and a miotic pupil. The iris is tan, with yellow pupillary margins and a thickened and vascular stroma.

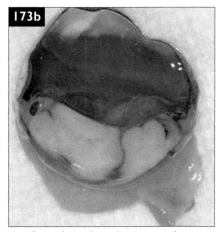

ii. The main differentials are anterior uveitis and uveal neoplasia. This is a cat with an invasive iris lymphosarcoma. Ocular ultrasound and aqueous centesis and cytology can aid diagnosis. Lymphosarcoma is the most common metastatic intraocular tumor in the cat.

iii. The level of pain and clinical appearance of iris tissue invasion led to enucleation of this globe. Histopathology confirmed iris lymphoma (173b, gross appearance of the iridal tumor). Systemic chemotherapy is recommended. Topical corticosteroids may reduce the size of the intraocular mass in the short term.

174 i. The cornea shows extensive vascularization with diffuse corneal edema (174a). A deep groove can be seen axially as well as a focal, round area of cellular infiltrate in the cornea. The conjunctiva is hyperemic with engorged blood vessels (174b). The clinical signs are consistent with chronic corneal ulcers.

ii. A foreign body was found embedded in the palpebral conjunctiva under the superior lid. Examination for foreign bodies under the lids and third eyelid should be performed in eyes with nonhealing ulcers. Other causes for chronic ulceration are distichia, ectopic cilia, trichiasis, entropion, keratoconjunctivitis sicca, and eyelid masses. Treatment varies according to the primary cause. In addition to elimination of the primary cause, treatment should include broad-spectrum topical antibiotics (determined by culture and sensitivity), as well as antiproteases (e.g. serum, EDTA, or N-acetylcysteine) and atropine. Systemic broad-spectrum antibiotics as well as anti-inflammatory drugs should be considered according to the severity of clinical signs.

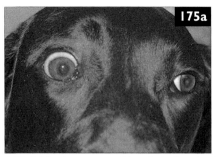
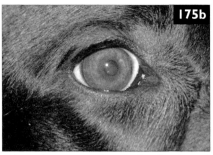

175 This three-year-old male Labrador Retriever is presented with dysphagia and 'strange-looking' eyes (175a, b). The owner reports that the dog is drooling excessively and having difficulty keeping food in his mouth. Examination reveals exophthalmos, a normal globe, and a reluctance to open the mouth.
i. What is your diagnosis?
ii. What is the pathophysiology of the disease?
iii. Why is the dog exophthalmic?
iv. What is the treatment for this condition?

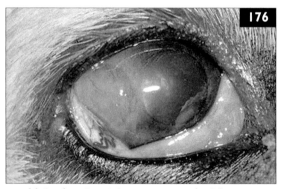

176 A three-year-old Cocker Spaniel was presented with a corneoscleral lesion at the nine o'clock position of the right eye (176).
i. Describe the lesion.
ii. What is your diagnosis, and is there a breed disposition?
iii. What are the pathogenesis and treatment for this disease?

175 i. Immune-mediated myositis of the masticatory muscles is the most likely diagnosis. Ultrasound and MRI were important in making this diagnosis.

ii. Immune-mediated myositis can have a general effect on skeletal muscle or be limited to the masticatory muscles. The muscles of mastication have a specific embryologic origin of their type 2 fibers that is associated with a unique type of myosin. In this disease, the immune system attacks the myosin of the masticatory muscles.

iii. Exophthalmos results from swelling of the inflamed muscles. As this disease progresses, the masticatory muscles atrophy and concomitantly fibrose, leading to an inability to open the mouth.

iv. As with most immune-mediated conditions, an immunosuppressive dose regimen of corticosteroids is the most effective treatment. With immune-mediated myositis it is imperative that treatment is initiated as soon as possible, as any muscle fibrosis that has already occurred is irreversible.

176 i. There is an elevated, pink, fleshy mass arising at the limbus and infiltrating the adjacent corneal stroma, with moderate corneal edema around the mass.

ii. Nodular granulomatous episcleritis (NGE). Nodular fasciitis, fibrous histiocytoma, proliferative keratoconjunctivitis, limbal granuloma, pseudotumor, and Collie granulomas are other terms for this disorder. Ocular findings in NGE include multiple, elevated, fleshy masses or a single mass arising at the limbus and infiltrating the adjacent corneal stroma. Nictitating membrane involvement is common, and there is a breed predisposition in the Collie, Cocker Spaniel, and Shetland Sheepdog. The lesions tend to be bilateral in the Collie and may tend to recur following therapy. In order to obtain a diagnosis, fine-needle aspiration or biopsy should be performed.

iii. The predominant histologic cell types in NGE are histiocytes, lymphocytes, and plasma cells. Production of lymphokines by the T lymphocytes and the resulting chemotaxis of histiocytes is a proposed pathogenesis of NGE. Generally, NGE tends to be benign clinically, with good response to oral azathioprine treatment in conjunction with topical administration of corticosteroids. Cyclosporin A can be used topically in conjunction with steroids initially, and then used alone to help prevent recurrence once the mass has resolved.

177 A two-year-old spayed cat was diagnosed with feline infectious peritonitis.
i. Describe the ocular findings (177).
ii. What is the pathophysiology of this process?

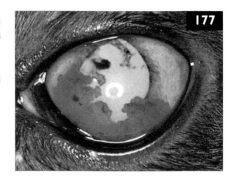

178 An adult cat presents with bilateral cataracts, with the left eye, shown here (178), being less advanced than the right.
i. Describe/name the cataract shown.
ii. What is a common cause of this type of cataract?

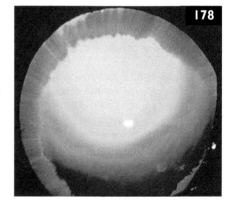

179 This photograph (179) depicts a small optic nerve head (ONH) from a young adult dog that has otherwise normal appearing eyes.
i. What is the diagnosis, and what does the pupil and pupillary light reflex (PLR) look like clinically in this patient?
ii. What is the vision of the eye of this dog?
iii. What breeds are predisposed to this condition?

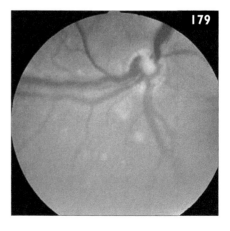

177 i. There are large, thick keratic precipitates (KPs), along with pigment and blood, adhered to the corneal endothelium at the ventral and medial cornea at the five to nine o'clock position. Fibrin is adherent to the anterior lens capsule and appears dark due to the retroillumination.

ii. KPs are accumulations of inflammatory cells, fibrin, and iris pigment. They are released due to blood–ocular barrier breakdown from vasculitis and/or vascular injury and deposited on the corneal endothelium. Convection currents in the aqueous humor aid this cellular distribution and attachment. In some granulomatous conditions (e.g. feline infectious peritonitis), KPs tend to form as large, waxy-yellow deposits, often called 'mutton-fat' deposits. These deposits are made of plasma cells and macrophages typical of granulomatous inflammation. KPs may partially resolve or be associated with permanent corneal opacification.

178 i. Linear, equatorial cataract. The nucleus is transparent.

ii. The equator is where new lens fibers are produced throughout life. The appearance of cataracts in this position suggests a recent change to the metabolism of the cat. The cat should be evaluated for diabetes and other metabolic diseases.

179 i. The optic disk is small and gray in color. There are no myelinated axons or nerve fibers noted on the disk. The retinal vasculature is normal, but looks large next to the small ONH. The diagnosis is micropapilla or optic nerve hypoplasia. These two terms are conditions that represent ranges of the same condition of reduced numbers of retinal ganglion cells. Micropapilla means the optic disk is smaller in size than average, but there is no effect on vision or the PLR. Optic nerve hypoplasia means there are significantly reduced numbers of retinal ganglion cell axons such that the optic nerve and optic disk are much smaller than the normal size. Eyes with optic nerve hypoplasia, as in this dog, would have a slightly dilated pupil and a slow PLR.

ii. The lack of retinal ganglion cells and their associated optic nerve axons would affect vision in this dog to some extent, but the dog may still have functional vision.

iii. Rough Collies, Beagles, Miniature Schnauzers, St. Bernards, Dachshunds, Shetland Sheepdogs, Irish Setters, German Shepherd Dogs, Cocker Spaniels, Standard Poodles, Miniature Poodles, Toy Poodles, Tibetan Spaniels, Soft-Coated Wheaten Terriers, Labrador Retrievers, Kerry Blue Terriers, Old English Sheepdogs, Afghan Hounds, Borzois, Golden Retrievers, Pharaoh Hounds, English Springer Spaniels, Keeshonds, Italian Greyhounds, Greyhounds, and Shih Tzus.

180 A spontaneous chronic corneal epithelial defect (SCCED) (Boxer ulcer) is shown (180a).
i. Describe the pattern of corneal neovascularization.
ii. Explain the pathogenesis of neovascularization.

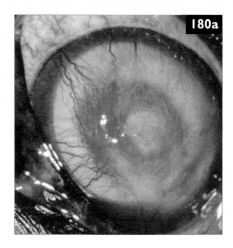

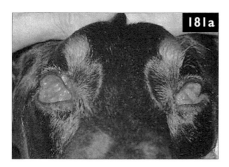

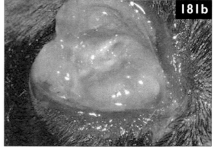

181 A two-year-old spayed female Doberman Pinscher is presented with severe conjunctivitis and a copious mucopurulent discharge (181a, b). The referring veterinarian believed that the globes were destroyed, but referred the dog for evaluation before enucleation. The same dog is shown after three months of medical therapy (181c).
i. What is the diagnosis?
ii. What is the pathogenesis of this condition?
iii. What is the treatment?

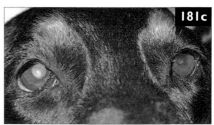

180 i. Superficial corneal blood vessels are growing from the limbus and forming large areas of pink granulation tissue at the center of the cornea.

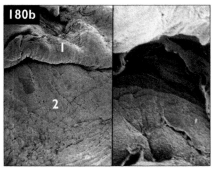

ii. Superficial vessels occur at the anterior third of the stroma and appear 'tree-like' or arborescent. They usually begin at the limbus as a single trunk vessel and branch extensively within the cornea. Very superficial vessels may be seen crossing the limbus because they are continuous with the conjunctival circulation. Deep intrastromal vessels are shorter and straighter, and branch less. They appear to arise from under the limbus because they are continuous with the ciliary circulation. Deep vessels suggest corneal stromal or intraocular disease, whereas superficial vessels are induced by surface (usually corneal epithelial) disease (180b, scanning electron micrograph of a superficial corneal ulcer involving primarily the anterior epithelium: 1, anterior epithelium; 2, corneal stroma). The image on the right shows the depth of the failed interaction/connection between the epithelium and the stroma. (See cases 8 and 64 for details of treatment of SCCED.)

181 i. Ligneous conjunctivitis.
ii. This is an idiopathic, breed-related, exuberant conjunctivitis of Doberman Pinscher dogs. The clinical presentation is dramatic, with proliferative conjunctivitis and ocular discharge. The palpebral conjunctiva and nictitating membranes are thickened and hyperemic with proliferative, opaque membranes. Affected dogs often display signs of concurrent systemic illness. Histopathologically, the affected conjunctiva has a thick, amorphous, eosinophilic, hyaline-like material in the conjunctival substantia propria, with a moderate mononuclear infiltrate. The surface of the conjunctiva is often encased in purulent debris and fibrin. The pathogenesis is unknown, but is speculated to be immune mediated. Congenital plasminogen deficiency can also occur in these dogs and may be part of the underlying cause of the ligneous conjunctivitis.
iii. Topical and subconjunctival administrations of fresh frozen plasma (FFP), topical administration of cyclosporin A, and oral administration of azathioprine have been used in some dogs. Excision of the membranes followed by intensive treatment with topical applications of heparin, tissue plasminogen activator, corticosteroid, and FFP, and intravenous administration of FFP prevented membrane regrowth in one case. Treatment was dramatically effective in this dog.

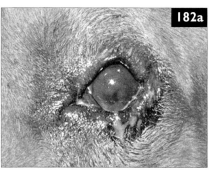
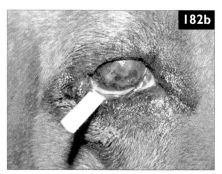

182 A dog has bilateral corneal disease (182a). The corneas are fluorescein negative.
i. What ophthalmic test is being performed in 182b?
ii. What disease process is present?
iii. What treatment options are available to improve the corneal disease in this dog?

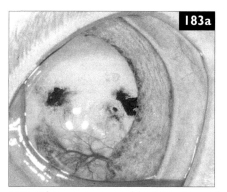
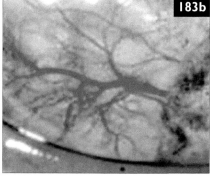

183 This seven-year-old white domestic shorthaired cat has been plagued with intermittent eye pain for several years (183a, b). There is no dazzle reflex or consensual pupillary light reflex to the other eye.
i. What is the most reasonable scenario for the lesions found in this eye?
ii. Is there any reasonable therapy for this eye?

182 i. Schirmer tear test (STT). A 5 by 35 mm strip is bent at the rounded tip and placed in the conjunctival fornix of the mid to lateral lower eyelid in contact with the cornea. Tears are allowed to migrate down the strip for 60 seconds. The strip is then removed and measured. Normal tear production is considered to be 15–25 mm wetting/min. Two types of STT can be considered. The STT I is performed without any topical anesthestic and measures reflex and basal tearing levels. The STT II is performed with topical anesthetic and measures only basal tear levels.
ii. Keratoconjunctivitis sicca (KCS, or 'dry eye'). There is yellow mucoid discharge on the cornea and eyelids. Pigment deposition on the corneal surface is present to such a significant degree that the anterior ocular structures (iris and pupil) cannot be visualized.
iii. Medical treatment modalities include topical immunomodulating medications (e.g. cyclosporin A [0.2% ointment or 1% and 2% solutions] and tacrolimus [0.03% ointment or solution]), topical antimicrobial and anti-inflammatory medications, and artificial tear replacement (see case **197**). In eyes with KCS and no corneal ulcers, topical corticosteroids are needed to reduce the conjunctivitis. Corticosteroids must be used with caution in eyes with KCS, as the corneal surface, being unhealthy from low tear levels, is more susceptible to corneal ulceration. There is a surgical option of parotid duct transposition available for KCS. For further examples of KCS see cases **42, 69, 94, 126,** and **199**.

183 i. This cat has chronic uveitis. A posterior synechia is present, with neovascularization of the lens from the iris. Uveal pigment has migrated onto the anterior lens capsule. The lens, which is mostly white, is now fully cataractous and most likely a result of the chronic uveitis. Dilatation of the pupil was not drug induced, but may have been caused initially by a retinal detachment. The posterior synechia has resulted in permanent mydriasis.
ii. Topical corticosteroids could help with eye pain. Enucleation is indicated if the pain is severe and cannot be controlled medically.

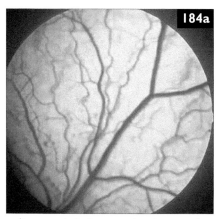

184 This (184a) is a direct ophthalmoscopic picture of a one-year-old Cocker Spaniel.
i. Describe the ophthalmoscopic findings.
ii. What is your diagnosis, and what is the etiology of this problem?
iii. What is the treatment?

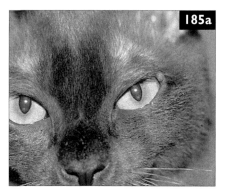
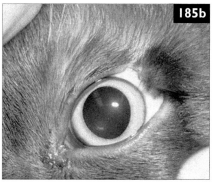

185 Two young Burmese cats were presented, each with a growth along the lateral canthus of the left eye. The growth in one cat was small and devoid of hair (185a). In the second cat the growth consisted of misaligned dark hairs attached to the bulbar conjunctiva near a defect in the lid margin (185b).
i. What are the masses associated with the conjunctivae and lids of these cats?
ii. What treatment(s) could be utilized to resolve the problem?

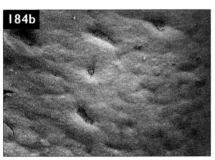
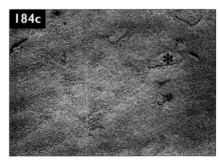

184 i. There are multiple, linear, retinal gray opacities in the tapetal region of the fundus.

ii. Retinal dysplasia, which is generally nonprogressive and does not usually interfere with vision. Retinal dysplasia has been defined as an anomalous differentiation of the retina. It is characterized histologically by folding of the sensory retina and formation of rosettes composed of retinal cells around a central lumen. As the sensory retina forms folds or raised areas, the outer segments of the photoreceptors elongate before pulling away from the underlying retinal pigmented epithelium (RPE) altogether, as seen in this scanning electron micrograph (184b). Concomitantly, the RPE forms extended microvilli and eventually disappears altogether (184c, asterisk indicates an area where the RPE has become totally disconnected from the sensory retina and the hexagonal shape of the cells is now visible). Spontaneous retinal dysplasia occurs in several breeds, and hereditary factors have been shown or suspected to be the cause in many. Multifocal retinal dysplasia has been reported in some breeds.

iii. There is no treatment. Dogs with retinal dysplasia should not be bred.

185 i. Congenital defects of the lateral canthus occur in Burmese cats and are associated with corneal and conjunctival dermoids. Nasal dermoids have also been observed in Burmese cats with eyelid dermoids.

ii. The lateral canthal defect is readily corrected surgically by excision and reconstruction of the lateral canthus. Conjunctival dermoids, as with most conjunctival neoplasms, are for the most part readily dissected away from the globe, being generally noninvasive.

186 This 12-year-old neutered domestic shorthaired cat was presented with blindness. Small hyperreflective lesions were seen ventrally (186a).
i. What is your diagnosis?
ii. What are the possible etiologies for this problem?

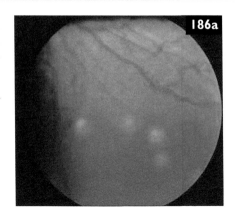

187 This is an eye (187) of an older male dog that had cataract surgery one year previously. What is seen in this eye?

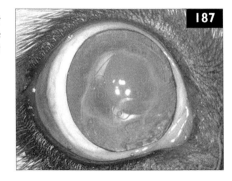

188 A specific technique is being performed on the upper eyelid region of this young Beagle in order to assess an ocular condition (188).
i. What technique is this?
ii. What feature is being assessed?
iii. How and why is this technique performed?

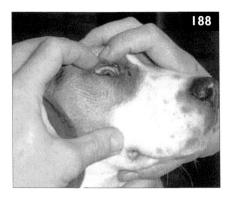

186 i. This is an active chorioretinitis. Chorioretinitis refers to inflammatory conditions that arise in the choroid and extend into the retina. The fuzzy outline to the lesions indicates retinal edema and activity (compare with case 67).
ii. Viral chorioretinitis in the cat has been associated with feline infectious peritonitis virus, feline immuno-deficiency virus, and feline leukemia

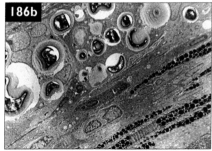

virus. Fungal chorioretinitis has been associated with cryptococcosis, histo-plasmosis, blastomycosis, coccidioidomycosis, and candidiasis. The protozoal agent *Toxoplasma gondii* is a documented cause of chorioretinitis in cats. Feline chorioretinitis and retinal detachment have been associated with tuberculous *Mycobacterium bovis*, as well as the nontuberculous agent *Mycobacterium simiae*. Parasitic infections such as dipteran larvae may cause chorioretinitis as the parasite migrates within or under the retina. In this case, *Cryptococcus* was identified as the cause of the chorioretinitis (186b, transmission electron micrograph of *C. neoformans* in the feline choroid). *C. neoformans* is the most commonly reported feline mycotic infection (see case 76).

187 An intraocular lens (IOL) has been placed in the lens capsular bag. The IOL is slightly out of position. Posterior capsular opacification surrounds the IOL. This opacification results from lens epithelial cell fibroplasia and is a common long-term complication of cataract surgery in dogs. This eye is still visual.

188 i. Digital tonometry.
ii. This form of tonometry is used to qualitatively assess the intraocular pressure (IOP) of the eye. Normal IOP in most animals is between 15 and 25 mmHg.
iii. To perform this diagnostic technique, the examiner stabilizes the globe with the fingers of one hand, while using the fingers of the other hand to apply gentle downward pressure along the lid margin. The accuracy of this procedure is dependent on the experience of the examiner; however, it is never as accurate as the quantitative objective measurement obtained from applanation tonometers (see cases 38 and 127).

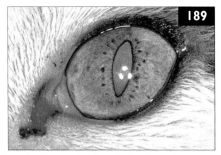

189 A nine-year-old male domestic shorthaired cat is presented with a two-week history of iris color change. On ophthalmic examination there is moderate aqueous flare, mild blepharospasm, and a miotic pupil (189).
i. What is the diagnosis?
ii. What are the differentials for this condition?
iii. What diagnostic tests should be considered?
iv. What is another typical clinical sign of this disease?
v. What are the treatment options?

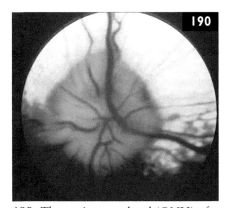

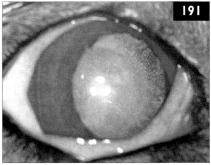

191 The eye of an 11-year-old mixed breed dog is shown (191).
i. Describe the ophthalmic findings shown.
ii. What are your clinical findings?

190 The optic nerve head (ONH) of a one-year old dog is shown (190).
i. What defines the shape of the ONH?
ii. Is the ONH in this dog normal or abnormal?

189 **i.** Anterior uveitis.

ii. Differentials include feline leukemia virus (FeLV), feline immunodeficiency virus (FIV), feline infectious peritonitis, toxoplasmosis, bartonellosis, cryptococcosis, histoplasmosis, coccidioidomycosis, blastomycosis, iris neoplasia, lens-induced uveitis, parasite migration, and idiopathic uveitis.

iii. Tests for FeLV and FIV should be submitted. This cat is positive for FIV.

iv. Cats with FIV-induced uveitis often have a pars planitis, which results in cellular infiltrates in the anterior vitreous and associated snowbanking or adhesion of these cells to the posterior lens capsule.

v. Supportive care for the FIV and treatment of the uveitis (see case **12**).

190 **i.** The prelaminar optic nerve is known as the optic disk, ONH, or optic papilla. Optic disk shape varies according to breed, the degree of axonal myelination, and the number of retinal ganglion cells. The canine optic disk has large prominent vessels that anastamose on the surface of the disk. There is often variation in disc diameter and shape of the canine ONH due to myelininated optic nerve axons anterior to the scleral lamina cribrosa. These cover the surface of the optic disk and continue into the retinal nerve fiber layer beyond the edge of the scleral canal such that the shape of the dog optic disk may be circular, triangular, or irregular. The canine ONH is white to pink in color, with a dark central spot called the physiological pit, a remnant of the hyaloid artery. In general, larger optic disks contain more nerve fibers than smaller disks.

ii. Normal.

191 **i.** There is pupil margin scalloping, nuclear lens opacity, and multiple, mobile vitreal opacities.

ii. Mild iris atrophy, nuclear sclerosis, and asteroid hyalosis, which are age-related ocular changes. Asteroid hyalosis is a form of vitreal degeneration and consists of conglomerates of calcium and lipids. Such opacities may move following movements of the globe. Vitreal degeneration may be age related, secondary to inflammation, or primary. Primary vitreous degeneration is also breed related and found in the Brussels Griffon, Chihuahua, Chinese Crested, Havanese, Italian Greyhound, Lowchen, Papillon, Shih Tzu, and Whippet.

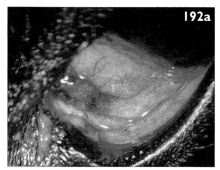

192 A three-month-old intact female American Cocker Spaniel was presented with significant unilateral epiphora. Flushing the superior punctum in the affected eye resulted in the formation of a bleb of tissue at the ventral punctum (**192a**).
i. What is the diagnosis?
ii. How can the diagnosis be confirmed?
iii. How is this condition treated?

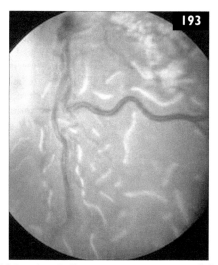

193 A four-week-old Border Collie puppy was presented for a general physical examination. The ophthalmic examination revealed the finding shown (**193**).
i. Describe this finding.
ii. What are the differential diagnoses, and how would you differentiate between them?

192 i. Punctal atresia, which may affect the superior, inferior, or both puncta. It can be either unilateral or bilateral and is commonly seen in American Cocker Spaniels, Bedlington Terriers, Golden Retrievers, Miniature and Toy Poodles, and Samoyeds.

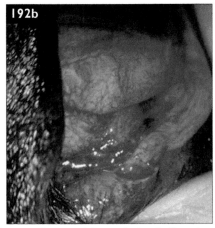

ii. Dorsal punctal atresia is asymptomatic and is diagnosed incidentally during routine biomicroscopic examination. Ventral punctal atresia is associated with epiphora in puppies, and confirmed by nasolacrimal flushing. The conjunctiva over the canaliculus will bulge during flushing.

iii. Ventral punctal atresia is treated by surgical excision of the ballooning conjunctiva (192b). The affected eye is then treated with topical antibiotic and corticosteroid solutions QID until re-examination in approximately seven days. If the punctum is patent and epiphora no longer present, further therapy is not required.

193 i. There are multiple, linear, retinal whitish opacities. The tapetum is blue due to the immaturity of this structure.

ii. This finding may be consistent with retinal dysplasia (see case 184) or with retinal folds. The high frequency of retinal folds among the eyes of puppies in some breeds, particularly the Collie and Shetland Sheepdog, has sometimes been interpreted as being a very mild form of retinal dysplasia. The folds are believed to result from the disparity of growth between the retinal layers and sclera, and they often resolve with growth and maturation of the eye. In contrast, retinal dysplasia represents abnormal differentiation of the retina and, therefore, would be expected to be permanent. Thus, a follow-up of these funduscopic alterations could indicate whether the lesions should be designated as retinal folds or retinal dysplasia.

194 A four-year-old male castrated cat is presented with a five-day history of blepharospasm, epiphora, and a red eye.
i. Describe the lesion shown (194).
ii. What is the most likely diagnosis?
iii. What are the treatment options?

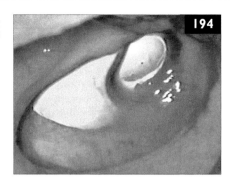

195 This dog (195) received the same surgical treatment as the dog in case 218. The image was taken one-year post operation.
i. What is happening in this instance?
ii. Why does this occur?

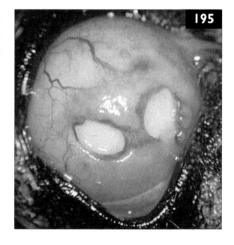

196 i. Describe the clinical signs shown in this dog (196).
ii. What is the diagnosis?
iii. What ocular changes can result from this condition if it becomes chronic?
iv. In this case it is already known that the cause for the eyelid condition was secondary to systemic adriamycin administration. In cases where the cause is unknown, how should this condition be worked up?

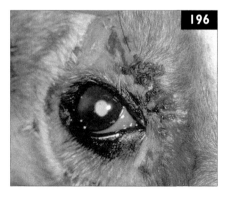

194 i. There is a moderate conjunctival hyperemia and a large-diameter, deep defect in the cornea. Some corneal vascularization is present and the pupil is dilated.
ii. A descemetocele. This is the deepest type of corneal ulceration, with corneal epithelium and stroma missing and exposure of Descemet's membrane (see case **232**). The membrane may bulge through the defect. To confirm the diagnosis of a true descemetocele, fluorescein stain should be applied, with gentle flushing after staining. The ulcer bed will stain positive at the ulcer edges, but not in the area where Descemet's membrane is exposed.
iii. Due to the risk of rupture, a descemetocele should be surgically repaired as soon as possible with a conjunctival flap, amnion graft, or corneal transplant. Direct suture closure of 1 mm diameter lesions can be attempted, but direct suturing is not recommended for large descemetoceles. Insertion of a donor corneal button or biosynthetic material into the defect will add strength to the cornea, and use of a conjunctival flap will both support the surgical area and aid vascularization.

195 i. A white intraocular prosthesis has eroded through the cornea and is now exposed.
ii. A corneal ulcer from infection or keratoconjunctivitis sicca could result in this problem. This breakdown occurred most likely due to mechanical irritation of the implant against the corneal endothelium and/or intraocular infection or contamination of the implant. The globe and implant were removed. (See also case **218**.)

196 i. Periocular crusts, hyperemia, and alopecia are present. The alopecia is noted in both eyelids and the crusting is mostly associated with the medial portion of the upper lids.
ii. Blepharitis.
iii. Corneal and conjunctival irritation associated with blepharitis may develop into entropion and/or ectropion. Scarring and infection of the eyelids may also develop due to self-trauma.
iv. Many cases of canine blepharitis, regardless of the cause, are infected. The infection may mask the initial cause of the blepharitis. Skin scrapings and skin biopsies with culture are important in the initial work-up for blepharitis. Systemic medications are critical to resolving eyelid inflammation. Further examples of blepharitis and their underlying causes can be seen in cases **77** and **210**.

197 A four-year-old cat is presented with a two-week history of a red squinty eye with a mucoid discharge (197a). The Schirmer tear test reading is 3 mm wetting/minute and there is a large superficial ulcer. One week later the cat is more uncomfortable and the cornea is melting (197b).
i. What is the most likely diagnosis?
ii. What are differentials for your diagnosis in a cat?
iii. What are the treatment options?
iv. What are the advantages of a conjunctival graft compared with a nictitans flap?

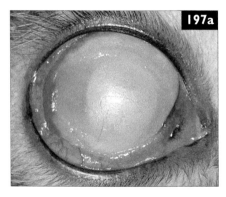

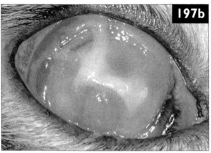

198 A two-year-old Portuguese Water Dog presents with optic neuropathy in both eyes (198).
i. Describe the findings shown in 198.
ii. What are causes of optic neuropathy?
iii. With what clinical signs might this dog present?

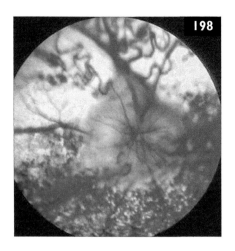

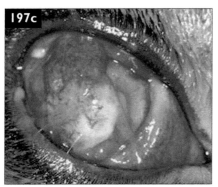
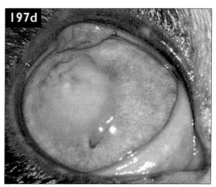

197 i. Keratoconjunctivitis sicca, with a secondary superficial ulcer.
ii. Differentials include blepharoconjunctivitis with lacrimal ductule obstruction and feline herpesvirus infection with chemosis of the lacrimal gland.
iii. Treatment options are aggressive medical therapy (see case **164**) and surgery. The surgical treatment of choice is a conjunctival graft (**197c**). The graft should be trimmed four weeks postoperatively to decrease scarring and increase the visual field (**197d**). Other options are amniotic membrane transplants and, in some cases, a nictitans flap.
iv. Conjunctival flaps provide structural support to the corneal lesion (more than a nictitans flap), provide blood vessels for stromal healing, provide a source of fibroblasts and connective tissue, and provide plasma from leaking vessels that may inhibit collagenase activity.

198 i. The optic disk is prominent, irregular in outline, and appears to be swollen due to obstructed axoplasmic flow. The blood vessels on the surface of the optic nerve head appear to be raised at the disk periphery. The retinal vessels are also tortuous. There are red focal perivascular areas of retinal hemorrhage.
ii. Optic neuropathies may be inflammatory or noninflammatory. Inflammatory optic neuropathies are termed optic neuritis and inflammation of the optic disk termed papillitis. Infection, reticulosis, and inflammatory orbital disease can cause optic neuritis. Swelling of the optic disk or papilledema can occur from elevated cerebrospinal fluid pressure. Glaucoma and optic nerve tumors cause optic disk swelling from obstructed axoplasmic flow. This dog's optic disks appear to represent a congenital problem. Function was normal.
iii. Fixed, dilated pupils and blindness. This dog's vision, pupillary light reflexes, and pupil size were, however, normal.

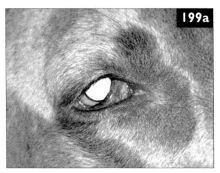

199 A two-year-old Weimaraner dog is presented with a one-week history of moderate conjunctivitis and mucoid ocular discharge (**199a**). The Schirmer tear test value is 0 for both eyes.

i. What are the differentials for absolute keratoconjunctivitis sicca (KCS)?

ii. On further examination, the dog's nose and gums are very dry. What is the most likely diagnosis?

iii. What are the treatment options?

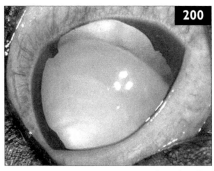

200 An eight-year-old Springer Spaniel is presented with a lens problem in the right eye (**200**).

i. Describe the clinical findings shown.

ii. What is the area with the yellow tapetal reflection in the upper portion of the photograph called?

iii. What anatomic structures that usually hold the lens in its normal position are compromised in this dog?

iv. What secondary complications may arise from lens luxation?

v. What is the surgical treatment for lens luxation?

199 i. Differentials for KCS in a young adult dog include neurologic KCS, drug-induced KCS, and autoimmune-mediated KCS.

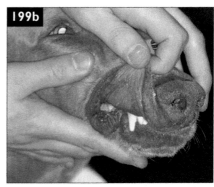

ii. Sjögren's syndrome, which is an autoimmune disease that attacks moisture-producing glands such as the tear and salivary glands. Sjögren's syndrome occurs in a small percentage of canine KCS patients. The clinical signs for this disease are KCS and a dry mouth due to lack of tears and saliva.

iii. Treatment options for absolute KCS (no tears at all) are limited to medical therapy. A parotid duct transposition will not be effective because of the lack of saliva in Sjögren's syndrome (**199b**). Medical therapy with topical immunosuppressive agents, such as cyclosporin A, tacrolimus, and/or pimecrolimus, is recommended, but may not be effective. Frequent application of topical ocular lubricant is helpful in preventing corneal ulceration and improving patient comfort.

200 i. There is moderate conjunctival hyperemia. The pupil is dilated and has irregular margins. Posterior synechiae are noted at seven and 10 o'clock. The lens is cataractous and posteriorly luxated, but is being held in position by the synechiae. The tapetal reflection can be seen dorsal to the lens.

ii. The aphakic crescent.

iii. The lenticular zonules must break to allow for the lens to become luxated. Reasons for zonular breakdown are discussed in case **236**.

iv. Secondary complications include inflammation, glaucoma, retinal detachment, and corneal endothelial damage.

v. Intracapsular lens extraction can be performed to remove the luxated lens. A 180 degree incision is made near the limbus from nine to three o'clock. The cornea is retracted, and the lens is extracted using a cryoprobe while detaching the vitreous from the posterior lens capsule with scissors. The corneal incision is then sutured closed.

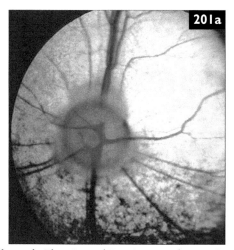

201 The fundus of a male Flat-Coated Retriever is shown (**201a**).
i. Is this fundus normal or abnormal?
ii. What is the name and origin of the dark spot in the center of the optic nerve head (ONH)?
iii. Which components of the ONH should be evaluated during eye examinations?
iv. What are the light tan, fuzzy appearing peripapillary areas?

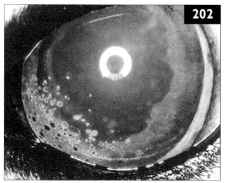

202 This seven-year-old mixed breed dog was presented for recheck five days after the beginning of medical therapy for canine ehrlichiosis.
i. What are the multiple, whitish, spherical opacities seen at the corneal endothelium (**202**)?
ii. With what other eye disease is the condition always associated?

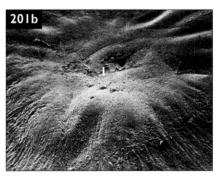

201 i. A normal fundus.
ii. A physiologic pit (see case 250). The physiologic pit is a remnant of the hyaloid artery (201b, scanning electron micrograph of a normal canine optic disk or nerve head with a remnant of the hyaloid artery [1]).
iii. The retinal vessels that anastamose on the optic disk surface, the neuroretinal rim (peripheral edge of the disk), and the optic cup (central disk area).
iv. The light tan fuzzy appearing lesion above the ONH is excess myelin in the retinal nerve fiber layer. This is a normal variation in some dog breeds.

202 i. Pigmented and nonpigmented keratic precipitates (KPs). A large area of iris depigmentation is also present.
ii. KPs are accumulations of inflammatory cells, fibrin, and pigment from the iris that are deposited on the corneal endothelium. It is important to note KPs because their presence is always indicative of uveitis. Topical anti-inflammatory therapy should be instituted immediately after the diagnosis of anterior uveitis is made. Failure to initiate therapy early in the disease process in cases of uveitis may result in many adverse sequelae, including synechiae formation, cataract, secondary glaucoma, endophthalmitis, and phthisis bulbi.

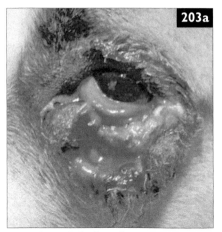

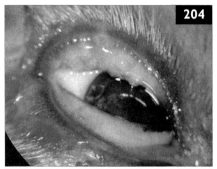

204 A six-month-old Golden Retriever is presented with swelling of the upper eyelid. When the conjunctiva is everted it appears to have small 'pustules' along the exposed, inflamed area (204). The puppy is blepharospastic and exhibits moderate tearing.
i. What is your diagnosis?
ii. Explain the disease and the consequences of the disease.
iii. How will you treat this condition?

203 This adult dog shown (203a) was presented with extensive lid laceration. What is the recommended therapy?

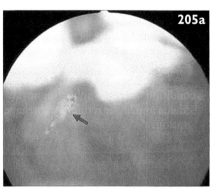

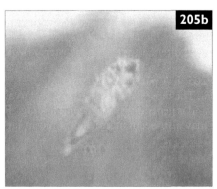

205 An object is seen in the vitreous in these fundus photographs of an eight-week-old Himalayan kitten (205a).
i. What is the linear structure (arrow in 205a and enlarged in 205b) floating in the vitreous?
ii. What is the most likely disease?

203 Eyelid lacerations are frequent in young small dogs and require surgical repair (203b). Both the wound in the lid and the conjunctival sac must be very thoroughly irrigated. Mechanical wound débridement should be kept to a minimum. Sutures at the eyelid margin should have their knots external to the free rim of the lid margin in order to avoid contact with the cornea. This can be accomplished with a figure-of-eight or cruciate suture. Two layers of sutures may be used in sterile wounds. The deeper palpebral conjunctiva and tarsus can be closed by simple continuous 6-0

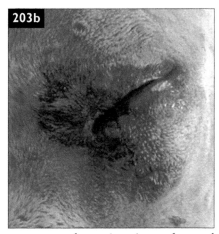

to 8-0 absorbable suture. Knots should not penetrate the conjunctiva surface and rub against the cornea. The skin, together with the orbicularis oculi muscle, is closed using simple interrupted nonabsorbable, 5-0 to 6-0 monofilament sutures. Absorbable material is used to close skin incisions in aggressive patients.

204 i. An inflamed meibomian or tarsal gland (also called meibomianitis).
ii. The meibomian glands produce the lipid part of the tear film. Meibomianitis is often secondary to bacterial infection and results in enlarged, painful, exudative meibomian glands. Meibomian gland adenitis can result in alterations of the lipid layer of the precorneal tear film and corneal ulceration. If meibomianitis becomes chronic, it can result in fibrosis and thickening of the eyelids and loss of the lipid secretion of the tear film.
iii. To provide the most accurate treatment, culture and sensitivity of the meibomian gland exudates is recommended. A topical and systemic broad-spectrum antibiotic and, often, a topical corticosteroid will be most effective in treating this condition.

205 i. A parasite.
ii. The most likely parasite is a fly larva. This condition is termed ophthalmomyiasis and is generally an incidental finding. Retinal edema and linear retinal hemorrhages may also be an indication of recent larval migration.

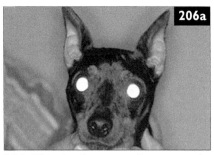

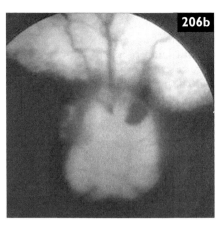

206 This dog has an optic neuropathy termed optic neuritis, which is caused by granulomatous meningoencephalitis (206a).
i. When a dog arrives at your hospital with blindness and fixed dilated pupils, what are the general disease processes that should be on the list of differentials?
ii. What diagnostic tests are performed to help identify the cause of the clinical signs associated with this patient?
iii. Describe what is seen in 206b.
iv. Define optic neuritis.
v. What are possible causes for optic neuritis in the dog?
vi. What is fluorescein angiography used to visualize?
vii. What abnormalities are being depicted in this fluorescein angiography image (206c)?

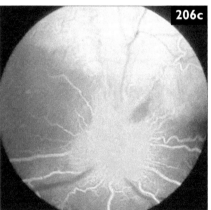

207 A five-year-old Boxer was presented with a six-month history of a red mass at the dorsal lateral limbus (207).
i. What is the most likely diagnosis?
ii. What are the treatment options?

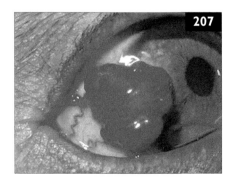

206 i. Optic nerve disease, retinal disease, visual cortex involvement, and glaucoma.
ii. Slit lamp biomicroscopy, indirect and direct ophthalmoscopy, and possibly electroretinography.
iii. The border of the optic nerve head (ONH) is less distinct and fuzzy due to edema or obstructed axoplasmic flow from nine to three o'clock. There is a focal area of hemorrhage at the one o'clock position on the ONH. The physiologic cup is indistinct and difficult to identify due to optic disk swelling.
iv. Optic neuropathies may be inflammatory or noninflammatory. Optic neuritis is inflammation of the optic nerve. A meningioma would cause a noninflammatory optic neuropathy.
v. Distemper, cryptococcosis, blastomycosis, ehrlichiosis, histoplasmosis, toxoplasmosis, head trauma, and orbital cellulitis are possible causes of optic neuritis in the dog. Neoplasia of the orbit or optic nerve, and optic nerve trauma from globe proptosis, toxins, vitamin A deficiency, and idiopathic optic nerve disease may have clinical signs resembling optic neuritis, but are noninflammatory in nature.
vi. The retinal and choroidal vasculature in order to evaluate the permeability of the vessels and to identify any pigment abnormalities.
vii. Swelling of the ONH. The optic disk hemorrhage that is noted in 206c is obstructing the fluorescence.

207 i. Hemangioma or hemangiosarcoma (see case 169). Hemangiomas and hemangiosarcomas are uncommon, but when they occur it is often at the lateral bulbar conjunctiva or the leading edge of the third eyelid. These tumors will invade the cornea and grow slowly in most cases, but some can be quite aggressive.
ii. The therapy of choice is a keratectomy and cryotherapy, laser ablation, or radiation. Depending on how large and deep the corneal defect is after keratectomy, a conjunctival or corneoscleral graft may be recommended. Enucleation may be required if the mass is large or has invaded the orbit. There have been no reports in dogs of metastasis of hemangioma or hemangiosarcoma from the eye to other organs.

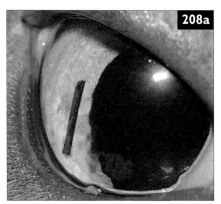

208 A young adult Siamese cat is presented with a filament-like object protruding from his eye (208a). What is the therapy for corneal foreign bodies as seen in this individual?

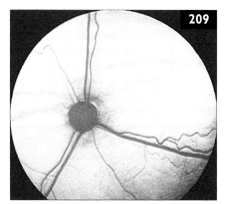

209 A middle-aged domestic shorthaired cat presents with this retinal lesion (209).
i. What caused the lesion in this cat?
ii. What stage of the condition is present?
iii. What are the etiology and pathophysiology?
iv. What is the therapy for this condition?

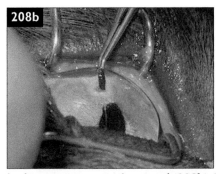

208 Corneal foreign bodies require surgical removal (208b). This can be as simple as using topical anesthetic and carefully flipping a superficial foreign body off the cornea with a cotton swab. Foreign bodies of the deep stroma or those that penetrate the anterior chamber will require general anesthesia and microsurgical techniques for surgical removal. Antimicrobials are recommended postoperatively.

209 i. This retinal lesion is typical of taurine deficiency retinopathy.
ii. The clinical presentation of taurine deficiency retinopathy in this case is relatively early, consisting of a horizontal band of hyperreflectivity dorsal to the optic nerve head.
iii. See case 22. Taurine is an essential amino acid for cats. The cones are initially affected in the entire retina, but early cone death is most easily detected in the area centralis, as noted in this photo, due to the high concentration of cone photoreceptor cells in this region.
iv. Taurine supplementation in the diet. The effects are only partially reversible and depend on the length of time the taurine deficiency has been present. Complete retinal degeneration is apparent after nine months if taurine is not supplemented.

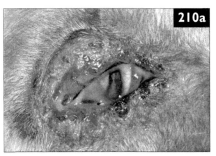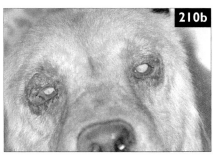

210 This adult male Labrador Retriever is presented with crusting and redness around the eyes (210a, b). The owner reports that this has recently worsened and that the dog has begun to traumatize himself by scratching and rubbing at the eyes. A moderate amount of purulent exudate is also present. Fluorescein staining is negative.
i. What is your diagnosis?
ii. What are the etiology and pathophysiology of this disease?
iii. What treatment do you recommend?

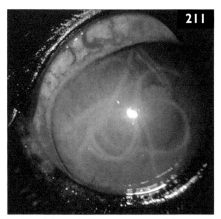

211 A three-year-old mixed breed dog presents with a two-day history of a red painful eye (211).
i. Describe the lesions.
ii. What is the etiology?
iii. What is the treatment?

210 i. Severe, bilateral blepharitis. Blepharitis is inflammation of the eyelids and is typically characterized by moderate to severe hyperemia, edema, and pain, which is indicated by severe blepharospasm (squinting) and excessive tearing. The condition is uncomfortable and the animal may subject himself to self-trauma.
ii. It is often difficult to determine the cause of blepharitis. Blepharitis can result from infectious causes (i.e. bacterial, mycotic, or parasitic) or it can be immune-mediated (for an in-depth review of causes and treatments see case 77). Due to the varied possible causes, the most effective way to diagnose the etiology of this condition is with a combination of tests. Skin scrapings and culture and biopsy of lid pyodermas are indicated.
iii. This was a bacterial blepharitis and it was treated with systemic antibiotics for two months.

211 i. There is moderate bulbar conjunctivitis and moderate corneal edema. Corneal vessels are present 360 degrees around the limbus. Multiple white curvilinear structures are present in the anterior chamber. The iris is swollen and the pupil dyscoric. When bright light is shone into the eye, these curvilinear structures exhibit motility.
ii. This patient has anterior uveitis due to heartworms. *Dirofilaria immitis* is the most commonly reported intraocular nematode among dogs in North America. Ocular involvement is postulated to be a result of aberrant migration of the fourth-stage larvae from the subconjunctival space. The parasites induce mild to severe anterior uveitis. In a retrospective study, German Shepherd Dogs were over-represented, with 33% of the study group affected.
iii. Surgical removal of the *D. immitis* worm through a limbal incision is generally successful. Preoperative treatment with a topical cholinesterase inhibitor may help to decrease parasite movement. After surgery, treatment for anterior uveitis is recommended (see case 12).

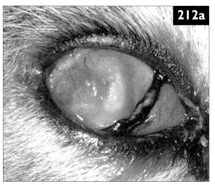
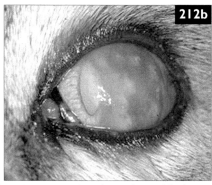

212 A three-year-old domestic shorthaired cat is presented with moderate blepharospasm and bilateral pink spots on both eyes of four weeks' duration (**212a, b**).
i. What is the most likely diagnosis for this case?
ii. What are two other differentials for this case?
iii. How is this disease diagnosed?
iv. What is the treatment for this condition?

213 This Rottweiler dog is presented with a large mass under the jaw (**213**). The owner is concerned about both the mass and the droopy looking right eyelid. Aspiration of the mass reveals a stringy, blood-tinged fluid with little to no cell population.
i. What are your differential diagnoses for this mass?
ii. What is the most likely diagnosis?
iii. What is the pathophysiology of the mass and the ectropion?
iv. How would you surgically correct the condition?

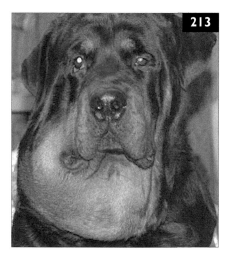

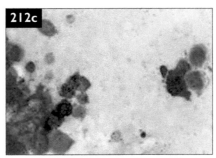

212 i. Eosinophilic keratitis (EK) occurs frequently in the cat. Ophthalmic examination usually reveals a localized-to-diffuse, white-to-pink granular appearing corneal plaque. Feline herpesvirus-1 has a strong link to EK, with 76% of cats with EK being feline herpesvirus-1 positive in one study.
ii. Differentials for a pink granular mass on the cornea in a cat are neoplasia (squamous cell carcinoma) and granulation tissue. It would be very rare to have either of these two differentials present bilaterally.
iii. Diagnosis of EK is based on cytology of corneal scrapings or histopathologic examination of corneal biopsies. Cytologic examination usually demonstrates the presence of eosinophils (**212c**), mast cells, lymphocytes, or plasmacytes.
iv. The treatment of choice when the corneal epithelium is intact is topical corticosteroids. Topical cyclosporin A can be useful in some refractory cases.

213 i. Differentials include sialocele and neoplasia (lymphoma, lipoma, salivary tumor).
ii. Based on analysis of the fine-needle aspirate, this dog has a large sialocele that is causing slight ectropion.
iii. The exact cause of sialoceles is unknown; however, trauma and foreign body penetration have been suggested. When the salivary gland is damaged, saliva leaks out into the surrounding tissue. Extravasated saliva then pools most commonly in the cranial cervical and intermandibular regions.
iv. Surgical drainage of the swelling and surgical removal of the sialocele are the treatments of choice. Following shrinkage of the sialocele, correction of the ectropion may be required, but was not necessary in this dog.

214 An 11-year-old intact male mixed breed dog was presented with a tan, flat, round mass on the lateral aspect of the upper eye lid (**214a**).
i. What is the likely origin of this mass, and what is the most likely diagnosis?
ii. How can this mass be treated?

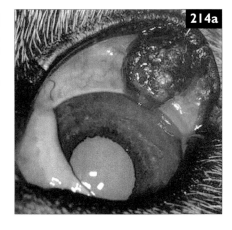

215 This domestic shorthaired cat was presented with the condition called iris bombé. Fibrin is present in the pupil and the anterior chamber is collapsed (**215**).
i. What is the mechanism for the formation of iris bombé?
ii. How is iris bombé treated?

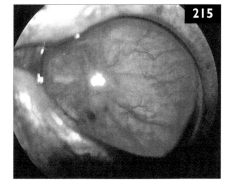

216 A 10-year-old male Golden Retriever is presented with bilateral painful red eyes. On ophthalmic examination there is mild conjunctival hyperemia, mild aqueous flare, and three to four blood-filled uveal cysts (**216**).
i. What is the diagnosis?
ii. What is its significance?

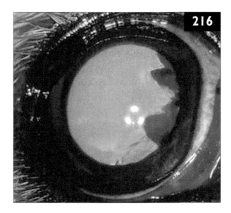

214 **i.** The mass is arising from the eyelid meibomian glands, so it is most likely an adenoma or adenocarcinoma. These tumors may be pink or have varying degrees of pigmentation, and are often lobulated. Some meibomian gland adenomas (**214b**) or adenocarcinomas may ulcerate and hemorrhage. They can cause blepharospasm, epiphora, conjunctival hyperemia, and corneal vascularization and pigmentation. Other tumors of the canine eyelids are melanomas, fibromas and fibrosarcomas, mastocytoma or mast cell sarcoma, lipomas, and papillomas.

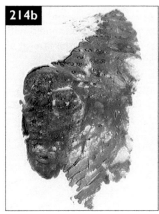

ii. Therapies for canine lid tumors include surgical excision, cryosurgery, or a combination of both. Recurrence rates after surgery and cryosurgery are low. Masses that involve the medial canthus and/or lacrimal puncta can be excised, but they are associated with damage to the nasolacrimal drainage system.

215 **i.** Chronic uveitis can lead to iris bombé. Miosis of the pupil is noted in response to prostaglandins and other inflammatory mediators that act directly on the iris sphincter muscle. Miosis causes increased iris lens contact to increase. Fibrin and inflammatory proteins released into the uveitic aqueous humor can cause rapid adherence or synechiation of the iris to the anterior lens capsule. If the synechiae occur for 360 degrees around the pupil, aqueous humor continues to be produced, which increases the pressure in the posterior chamber and pushes the iris anteriorly to narrow the anterior chamber. Glaucoma is a result of iris bombé.

ii. Medically. The uveitis is suppressed with topical corticosteroids and attempts to dilate the pupil are made with topical atropine and phenylephrine. Tissue plasminogen activator is used in acute cases in an attempt to breakdown the fibrin causing the synechiae. The prognosis is poor for vision if iris bombé remains.

216 **i.** Pigmentary uveitis. Clinical signs of this condition are radially oriented pigment on the anterior lens capsule, multifocal pigmented iris areas with or without uveal cysts, blood-filled uveal cysts, spiderweb-like fibrinous debris in the anterior chamber, and posterior synechiae.

ii. Pigmentary uveitis is a progressive blinding disease in the Golden Retriever. Medical therapy for uveitis should be started immediately and will be long term (see case **12**). Complications are glaucoma and cataracts, with both likely to cause blindness.

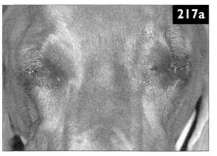 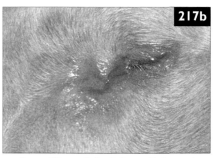

217 A young Weimaraner presents with a soft swelling of the left medial canthus (**217a, b**).
i. Describe the clinical signs seen in this dog.
ii. What is the most likely diagnosis?
iii. What clinical sign will be noted in all patients with this condition?
iv. What is the treatment for this type of condition?

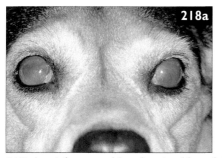 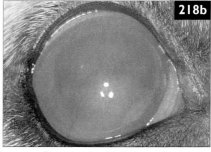

218 An eight-year-old male mixed breed dog was diagnosed with bilateral primary glaucoma that left the dog permanently blind. The chosen therapy was an intraocular prosthetic placement. The two images shown were taken one year postoperatively (**218a, b**).
i. Why do you suspect intraocular prostheses were chosen as therapy in this dog?
ii. Do the eyes look as expected one-year postoperatively?

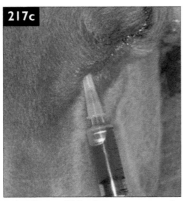

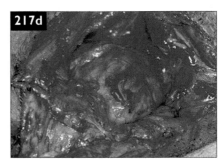

217 i. Bilateral blepharospasm and epiphora are noted. There is a swelling medial and ventral to the medial canthus of the left eye (**217b**). It is possible that a similar lesion (although smaller) may exist in the same location in the right eye.

ii. A canaliculops, a congenital cyst of canalicular origin. The lacrimal drainage system of the dog consists of a lacrimal punctum in the upper and lower lids. These each connect to a lacrimal canaliculum and they merge to form a single naso-lacrimal duct that drains into the nose.

iii. Epiphora is noted secondary to compression of the canaliculi by the canaliculops.

iv. The cystic fluid can be removed using a syringe and needle (**217c**). This may improve the clinical signs temporarily, and the fluid can be used for diagnostic purposes. Surgical removal of the cyst (**217d**) can restore canalicular patency and therefore improve the patient's epiphora.

218 i. Long-term intraocular pressure (IOP) elevation leads to retinal damage and blindness. When blindness occurs, enucleation or intraocular prosthetics would be recommended. Some owners prefer the cosmetic appearance of prostheses, although the dogs surely do not care! The dogs are no longer painful and do not require expensive IOP reducing medications after enucleation or prosthesis implantation. Prosthetic placement should not be done if the dog has keratoconjunctivitis sicca or corneal degeneration, or if the glaucoma was caused by intraocular infection or neoplasia.

ii. Following placement of an intraocular prosthesis, the globe will shrink around the implant and the cornea will vascularize and become gray. The dark color is the result of the globe color combined with the black color of the prosthesis.

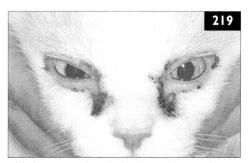

219 A three-year-old domestic shorthaired cat is examined and found to have blepharospasm, epiphora, and moderate conjunctivitis (219). The cat has just moved to a new house.
i. What is the most likely diagnosis?
ii. What is the cause of the brown tear staining?
iii. Why are the eyes different colors?

220 This 12-year-old dog was presented with mild, painless exophthalmos of the left eye.
i. Describe the findings of the ophthalmoscopic examination (220a) and ultrasonogram (220b).
ii. What is your differential diagnosis and treatment?

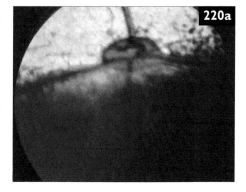

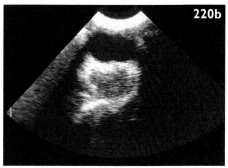

219 i. Herpes conjunctivitis (see case **31**). Feline herpesvirus-1 (FHV-1) becomes latent in the trigeminal ganglia and will recrudesce when the cat is stressed. Severe ocular surface inflammation from FHV-1 infection in kittens may cause acquired punctal stenosis or occlusion. Symblepharon (abnormal adhesion of the bulbar and palpebral conjunctivae) can obliterate one or both of the punctal openings. To confirm occlusion, careful examination of the punctal opening under magnification can be performed.
ii. The brown tear staining is caused by a lactoferrin-like pigment in the tears. Tear staining is often seen in white-coated animals, but it does occur in dark-coated animals as well. Bacterial action on the tear proteins can exacerbate the amount of staining.
iii. This cat has iridal heterochromia, or two different iris colors. This can be a normal finding, as in this cat, or be secondary to anterior uveitis or iris melanomas.

220 i. The ophthalmoscopic examination shows deformation and indentation of the ventral edge of the optic nerve head; the ultrasonogram indicates a space-occupying structure in the orbit.
ii. Orbital tumors and abscesses should be considered in the diagnosis. Tumors represent the most common group of orbital diseases. The most frequent orbital neoplasms are fibroma, meningioma, osteosarcoma, and lymphosarcoma. Orbital tumors are mostly primary and malignant. As expected, all kinds of tumors occur. Orbital tumors cause slowly progressive unilateral exophthalmos, with variable displacement of the globe, while orbital abscesses are generally acute in onset and very painful. In contrast to orbital inflammatory diseases, orbital neoplasms are not initially painful. Ultrasonography and, preferably, CT or MRI can demonstrate the extent of orbital neoplasia and careful fine-needle aspiration can be used to make a definitive diagnosis. Surgical removal of the neoplasm is performed in localized masses, ideally with preservation of the globe and vision. If preservation of the globe is not possible, exenteration of the globe or radical orbitectomy must be considered. Surgical management of orbital neoplasia can be combined with radiation therapy, chemotherapy, or both. In most cases the prognosis is guarded at best. Fine-needle aspiration revealed orbital lymphosarcoma in this dog.

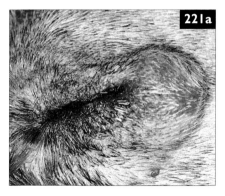

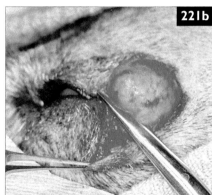

221 You are presented with a 10-year-old mixed Terrier that is exhibiting redness and alopecia associated with a lateral canthal mass of the left eye (221a). Surgical removal of the mass (221b, c) and biopsy reveal a chondroma.
i. What would have been your differential diagnoses for a lateral canthal mass?
ii. What are the etiology and pathophysiology of chondromas?
iii. Discuss the surgical procedure for removal of this mass.

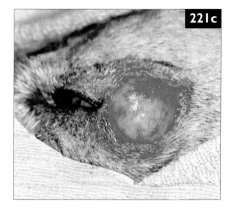

222 This fundus photograph (222) was taken from a 15-year-old domestic shorthaired cat.
i. Describe the clinical findings.
ii. What ocular abnormalities are associated with systemic hypertension in the cat?
iii. The blood vessel located at 12 o'clock has successive dilatations, referred to as 'boxcars'. What is the pathophysiology of the clinical sign of 'box carring'?

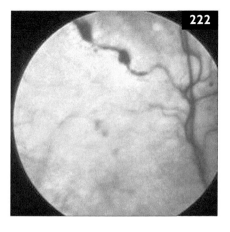

207

221   i. Chondroma, sebaceous adenoma/adenocarcinoma, squamous cell carcinoma, melanoma, or other neoplasms.
ii. Chondromas are tumors associated with cartilaginous tissues.
iii. Surgical excision followed by reconstructive blepharoplasty will be required to remove the mass and achieve acceptable cosmesis. The skin around the mass must be dissected away and removed. A lateral canthoplasty and dissection around and under the mass to determine the extent of its attachment are required for complete removal. Reconstructive blepharoplasty can be performed on the lateral canthus following mass removal using the Z-plasty procedure (as described in various textbooks).

222   i. There is a segmental constriction and dilatation of blood in the vessels. This is termed 'box carring'.
ii. Retinal hemorrhage, 'box carring', retinal detachments, retinoschisis, retinal edema, retinal degeneration, hyphema, and glaucoma.
iii. Hypertension can lead to sustained vasoconstriction of the retinal arterioles, which can result in ischemic damage and degeneration of the retina. Red blood cells and plasma leak from vessels into the retinal tissue when endothelial cells and vascular smooth muscle become compromised and this causes very high increases in the tissue pressure. This is visualized as retinal hemorrhage, retinal edema, and retinoschisis. 'Box carring' is caused by the retinal tissue pressure being higher than the intravascular pressure such that the vessels collapse in certain segments. The intravascular pressure then builds up and forces blood forward until it reaches a new point, where the vessel again collapses and the process begins again. Note how this process differs from that seen in case **244**, which also involved ocular hypertension in the cat.

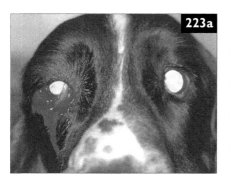

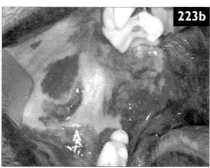

223 Exophthalmos associated with orbital neoplasia was present in this English Springer Spaniel (223a). An abscess was drained behind the last molar tooth (223b). A drain was placed to aid removal of the exudate (223c).

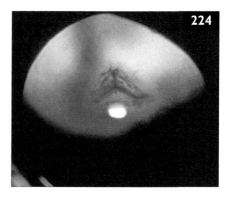

i. What clinical signs are associated with orbital neoplasia?
ii. What other orbital neoplasms have been identified in domestic species?
iii. Approximately what percentage of canine orbital tumors are malignant?
iv. What is the recommended surgical approach to removal of an orbital neoplasm?
v. What follow-up therapy may be recommended after surgical removal of the tumor is performed?

224 A two-year-old female Golden Retriever presents for her annual vaccinations. On ophthalmic examination a cataract is discovered (224).
i. Describe the cataract.
ii. Is this cataract going to progress to blindness?
iii. Should the client breed this dog?
iv. What is the treatment recommendation?

223 i. Unilateral exophthalmos (which is usually painless), reduced motility of the globe, deviated globe, protrusion of the third eyelid, exposure keratitis secondary to exophthalmos, periocular swelling, dilated pupil, nasal discharge, and blindness. This dog had an orbital squamous cell carcinoma that was necrotic and thus had some degree of pain.

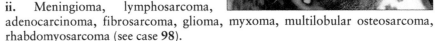

ii. Meningioma, lymphosarcoma, adenocarcinoma, fibrosarcoma, glioma, myxoma, multilobular osteosarcoma, rhabdomyosarcoma (see case **98**).

iii. About 80–90%.

iv. An exploratory orbitotomy by zygomatic arch resection. Resection of the tumor can be attempted, but orbital exenteration may be necessary.

v. Radiation therapy (**223d**), chemotherapy, or immunotherapy. In this case, iridium implants controlled the condition for over a year.

224 i. This is a posterior triangular suture line cataract. The cataract is in the posterior part of the lens because the posterior Y suture is an upside down Y. This is the typical location (posterior subcapsular cataract) for a breed-related cataract in Golden Retrievers and Labrador Retrievers.

ii. In rare cases the cataract will slowly progress to maturity and cause blindness. There is a second breed-related cataract in the Golden Retriever that is a progressive cortical cataract.

iii. There is most likely an autosomal-recessive mode of inheritance in both the Golden and Labrador Retriever. It has been suggested that the triangular cataracts are heterozygotes and the more progressive cataracts are homozygotes. In order to reduce the spread of inherited cataracts in this breed, it is recommended that the dog is not bred

iv. Fortunately, this breed-related cataract rarely progresses, but it should be monitored yearly. There is no preventive medical or surgical treatment for cataract formation.

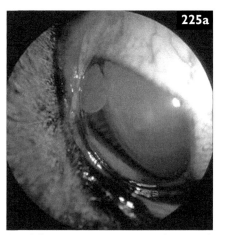
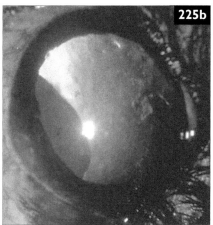

225 These two images (225a, b) are taken from two dogs, each with a ciliary body mass.
i. Describe the clinical appearance of these two dogs.
ii. What is the most likely diagnosis?
iii. What other lesions are likely to be on the differential list when clinically evaluating masses in this location?
iv. What type of stains used on this tumor tissue are retained?

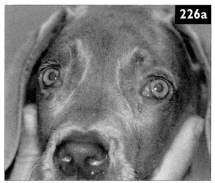
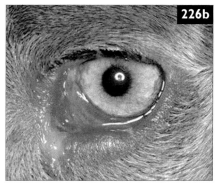

226 Severe conjunctivitis is present in this two-year-old dog (226a, b).
i. Describe the clinical signs noted in these photographs.
ii. What is the association between this orbital disease and conjunctivitis in dogs?
iii. What other clinical signs may also be noted with this orbital condition?

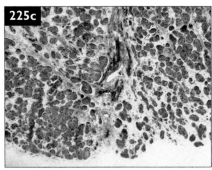

225 i. In both photographs there is a pink fleshy mass located posterior to the pupillary margin through a dilated pupil.

ii. Ciliary body adenomas, which are the most common tumors of the ciliary body and iris, and comprise the second most common intraocular tumor of the dog. The epithelial tumors become distinctly gland-like in their appearance (225c).

iii. Melanomas have a similar clinical presentation and location. Uveal cysts should also be considered.

iv. Vimentin, S100, neuron-specific enolase, and Alcian blue will all stain positive.

226 i. There is epiphora of the ventral eyelid. A mild light yellow mucoid discharge is noted at the medial canthus. Severe hyperemia of the conjunctival surface of the third eyelid is visible. The conjunctiva appears necrotic in some areas and there is protrusion of the left third eyelid. The dog has been diagnosed with sinus osteomyelitis.

ii. Orbital cellulitis and conjunctivitis can be seen with sinus disease. The conjunctiva is commonly the first ocular tissue to show irritation, swelling, or displacement in orbital and sinus disease.

iii. Fistulous tracts, blepharedema, and exophthalmos.

227 This eight-month-old Dachshund was presented with chorioretinitis caused by a *Coccidioides* sp. infection (227).
i. What is the organism that causes coccidioidomycosis in dogs?
ii. How is this disease spread?
iii. In what regions is coccidioido-mycosis more common?
iv. What are the ocular manifestations of coccidioidomycosis?
v. How can the diagnosis of cocci-dioidomycosis be made?
vi. What systemic treatments can be used for coccidioidomycosis?

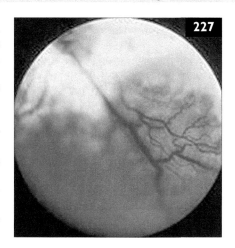

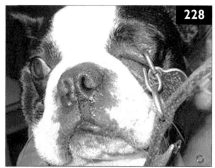

228 A six-year-old spayed female Boston Terrier was presented with a traumatic foreign body (tag hook with collar attached) in the upper eyelid (228).
i. What should be done before removing the foreign body?
ii. What are the treatment options?
iii. What is the postoperative care?

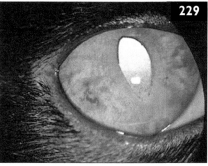

229 A young domestic shorthaired cat has feline infectious peritonitis (FIP) and presents with this iris disease (229).
i. What form of FIP is more often associated with ocular lesions?
ii. What is the most common ocular manifestation of FIP, and what clinical sign is being depicted in the cat in 229?
iii. What causes FIP, and what are other ocular manifestations of this disease?

213

227 i. *Coccidioides immitis* is a spherical dimorphic saprophytic fungus that lives in soil.
ii. The organism is spread through inhalation of the fungal spores.
iii. This disease is endemic in low altitude areas of the southwestern United States. It is also seen in Mexico and Central and South America.
iv. Granulomatous uveitis and iritis are associated with the anterior segment, and chorioretinitis and retinal detachment are associated with the posterior segment.
v. Vitreocentesis and anterior chamber centesis could yield fungal elements. PCR has been developed to identify the DNA of the organism, but it can be of limited help due to the short-term duration of the DNA within the serum of the dog. Latex agglutination, agar gel immunodiffusion, and ELISA have been used for identification, as well as complement fixation titer and measuring IgG antibodies.
vi. Ketoconazole, itraconazole, or fluconazole. Treatment is of long duration.

228 i. An ophthalmic examination should be performed. The cornea and anterior chamber should be carefully examined. Corneal laceration and perforation are potential complications to lid trauma. The anterior chamber should be examined for hyphema, lens material, and pupil size.
ii. Eyelids are highly vascular and have a great capacity to heal and resist infection. The treatment of choice is removal of the tag hook and primary closure of the wound. Alternatively, the hook can be cut and removed under sedation, and the wound allowed to heal by second intention.
iii. Postoperative care includes topical and/or systemic antibiotics, systemic anti-inflammatories (e.g. carprofen), and an Elizabethan collar. Ice packs immediately postoperatively and warm compresses 2–4 days postoperatively can reduce lid swelling.

229 i. The noneffusive or dry form of FIP.
ii. Granulomatous anterior uveitis with large mutton-fat keratic precipitates and fibrin in the anterior chamber is commonly found in the eyes of cats with FIP. Rubeosis iridis (iris neovascularization) is seen in this cat.
iii. FIP is a coronavirus. Chorioretinitis is also found in cats with with FIP. A pyogranulomatous exudate may be located perivascularly in retinal vessels. There may also be retinal detachments, optic neuritis, and retinal hemorrhages.

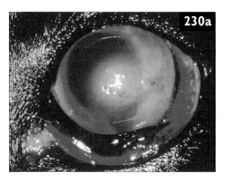

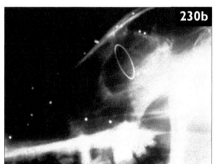

230 An adult mixed breed dog was presented with wounds consistent with those inflicted from a shotgun blast. Corneal perforation from a steel pellet is seen (230a). Radiography (230b, c) is performed.
i. Discuss the radiographic findings.
ii. What other imaging technques might be useful?

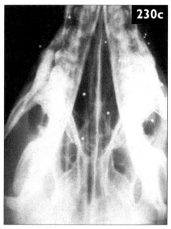

231 A nine-year-old dog presents with a one-week history of painful red eyes (231). The dog has bilateral severe anterior uveitis and a swollen iris. On physical examination there is lymph-adenopathy.
i. What diagnostic test should be performed?
ii. What is the diagnosis?
iii. What are the treatment options?
iv. What is the prognosis?

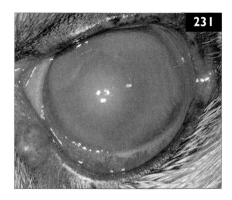

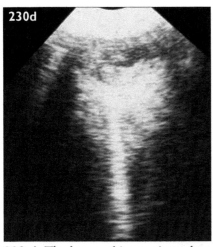

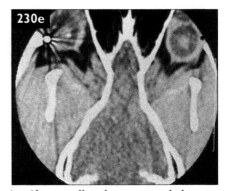

230 i. The key to this case is to determine if any pellets have entered the eye. Metallic objects can be seen in several places in the radiographs, but the plain films do not determine if the pellets are intraocular or not.

ii. Ultrasound (the ultrasonogram [230d] shows a reverberation artifact as the pellet blocks the soundwaves from the ultrasound probe) and CT (the 'starburst sign' [230e] localizes the pellet to inside the globe). An MRI should not be used for the localization of metallic foreign bodies, as the magnet could indiscriminately pull the pellet out of the globe, resulting in further trauma.

231 i. Fine-needle aspiration of the lymph nodes should be performed.

ii. Cytology of the lymph node revealed lymphosarcoma (see case 173). Lymphosarcoma is the second most common intraocular neoplasia in dogs. Ocular disease can be the presenting complaint and is often bilateral. A large prospective study revealed that 37% of lymphosarcoma patients present with some ocular lesions.

iii. Medical therapy for anterior uveitis should be started immediately (see case 12). Enucleation of the globe does not improve survival time, but may improve quality of life due to elimination of the ocular pain caused by uveitis and secondary glaucoma. For treatment options for lymphosarcoma, current internal medicine textbooks should be consulted.

iv. Poor. Most animals with ocular lymphoma lesions are in the advanced stages of lymphoma and may also have leukemia. The survival times for dogs with ocular lymphoma are short.

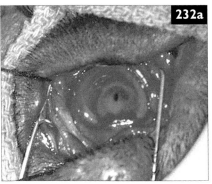
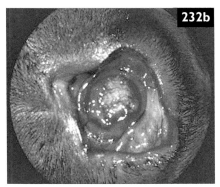

232 A four-year-old Coonhound is presented with a small descemetocele and corneal ulcer in the axial cornea.
i. What surgical method has been used to treat the descemetocele (232a, b)?
ii. What are the cons and pros for this procedure compared with the alternative ones?

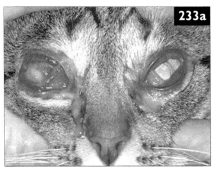
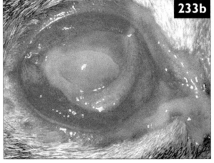

233 A 12-year-old domestic shorthaired cat is presented with a two-week history of red squint eyes (233a, b).
i. Describe the lesions.
ii. What are the differentials for the conjunctival lesions?
iii. What are the differentials for the corneal lesion in the right eye?

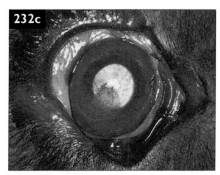

232 i. A conjunctival free island graft.

ii. A conjunctival free island graft is a modified conjunctival graft as it has no blood supply. These grafts are essentially a transplant of conjunctival tissue to the cornea for deep corneal ulcers or corneal perforations. The success of this surgical procedure may depend on the vascularity of the lesion, therefore lesions without corneal vascularization may heal better with a typical conjunctival pedicle graft. The advantages of the free island grafting procedure are: tissue is readily available; a watertight, 360° closure can be made; there is no tension to cause premature retraction of the graft: and the graft does not require trimming after surgery as do conjunctival pedicle or bridge flaps. The eye is shown four weeks postoperatively (232c).

233 i. There is bilateral severe conjunctival hyperemia and chemosis. The conjunctiva is thickened. The left cornea is clear and a green tapetal reflection is observed. The right cornea has no tapetal reflection; there is a tan to pink gelatinous raised oval-shaped central lesion and corneal vascularization with edema.

ii. The differentials include viral (feline herpesvirus-1) and bacterial (e.g. *Chlamydophila*, *Myoplasma*) infection, meibomian gland adenitis, keratoconjunctivitis sicca, eosinophilic keratoconjunctivitis, conjunctival trauma or foreign body, and neoplasia. This was a case of conjunctival lymphosarcoma.

iii. The differentials include descemetocele, corneal foreign body, iris prolapse, melting corneal ulcer, epithelial inclusion cyst, corneal endothelial dystrophy, and sloughing corneal sequestrum. This was a case of iris prolapse.

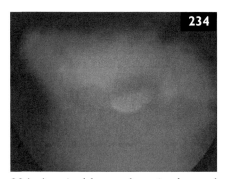

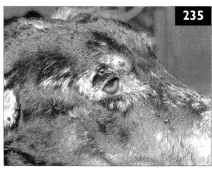

234 A retinal hemorrhage is observed (234) during funduscopic examination of a middle-aged male mixed breed dog.
i. Where is this retinal hemorrhage, called 'keel boat', located in relation to the retina?
ii. What type of disease processes may have 'keel boat' hemorrhages as a clinical sign on ophthalmoscopic examination?
iii. Describe the other types of retinal hemorrhage that can be visualized on ophthalmoscopic examination, and the location that corresponds to the shape.

235 A six–year-old male Doberman Pincher is presented with a four-week history of vitiligo (depigmentation of the skin) around his eyes (235).
i. What are the differentials for depigmented skin around the eye?
ii. There is no generalized vitiligo, but no detectable uveitis. What is the most likely diagnosis?
iii. What is the pathogenesis of the skin lesions?

236 A six-year-old mixed breed dog presents with a two-day history of a painful eye. On ophthalmic examination a crescent-shaped structure is seen behind the pupil (236).
i. Describe the lesion.
ii. What is the diagnosis?
iii. What is the pathophysiology of this condition?
iv. What are the treatment options?

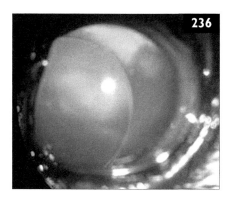

234 i. The hemorrhage is preretinal and is located in the vitreous in front of the retina. The superficial retinal vessels can leak and cause separation of the vitreous from the retina and, in association with gravity, the shape of the hemorrhage is that of a 'keel boat', as its rounded end points toward the six o'clock position.
ii. This type of hemorrhage may be associated with infectious chorioretinitis from rickettsial diseases and from systemic hypertension.
iii. Subretinal hemorrhages, which are located between the retina and the choroid, appear as large areas of indistinct bordered, diffuse, dull-red areas of hemorrhage. Superficial retinal hemorrhages, located within the nerve fiber layer, are visualized as linear brush or flame shapes. Hemorrhages located in the deep retina are usually visualized as small, discrete, round hemorrhages.

235 i. Differentials include zinc deficiency, lupus erythematosus, and uveodermatologic syndrome.
ii. The immune-mediated disease lupus erythematosus. Discoid lupus erythematosus is limited to the skin, and systemic lupus erythematosus is a multiorgan disease. Both forms frequently have a facial dermatosis with eyelid involvement.
iii. The pathogenesis of the skin lesions involves an autoimmune response where antinuclear antibodies bind to the keratinocytes. The antibodies then cause cytotoxic injury and cytokine release, resulting in attraction of lymphocytes and epithelial damage. A current internal medicine text will help with the details of diagnosis and treatment.

236 i. The cornea is clear and there is an aphakic crescent to the right as the lens is luxated to the left. A clear view of the optic nerve, tapetum, and nontapetal region can be seen to the right in the aphakic crescent.
ii. Lens luxation.
iii. The pathophysiology of lens luxation is unknown. An inherited defect in the suspensory apparatus or ciliary zonules of the lens is the cause of primary lens luxations in terrier breeds and Shar Peis. Inflammatory cells may attack the zonular fibers in dogs with a lens luxation and anterior uveitis. Buphthalmia as a result of glaucoma will also cause lenses to either subluxate or fully luxate into the anterior chamber or vitreous.
iv. Treatment options are both medical and surgical (see case **62**).

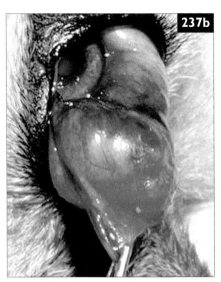

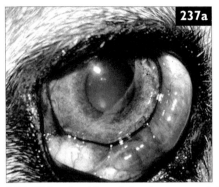

237 This mixed breed dog is presented for recent development of a mass external to the globe (237a, b). The owner said it occurred suddenly and she was afraid it might be cancer. Careful manipulation of the mass reveals a soft, pigmented, 'oily' mass loosely attached to the globe.

i. What are your differential diagnoses?
ii. Describe how you might quickly determine the etiology of the mass?
iii. What is the treatment for this condition?
iv. What is the prognosis?

238 A seven-year-old mixed breed dog is presented with bilateral moderate blepharitis and loss of periocular hair of two weeks duration (238).
i. What diagnostic test should be performed?
ii. What are the differentials for canine blepharitis?
iii. This patient also has truncal alopecia, weight gain without an

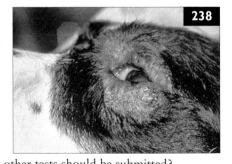

increase in appetite, and dry skin. What other tests should be submitted?

237, 238: Answers

237 i. Possible differentials include cherry eye (prolapse of the nictitating gland), third eyelid neoplasia (lymphoma, lipoma, sarcoma, melanoma), and orbital fat prolapse.
ii. A fine-needle aspirate of this mass found a large number of adipocytes, so a diagnosis of orbital fat prolapse was made.
iii. Orbital fat prolapse occurs due to breakdown of the orbital septum. It is treated surgically by removal of the prolapsing fatty tissue followed by suturing of the conjunctiva to the episcleral tissue.
iv. Recurrences can occur.

238 i. All dogs with blepharitis should have a Schirmer tear test (STT) performed (see case 113). This dog has a STT value of 5 mm wetting/minute, indicating significant keratoconjunctivitis sicca (KCS). Dogs with blepharitis should also have skin cytology and/or histology performed.
ii. Differentials for bilateral blepharitis are bacterial (staphylococci and streptococci), mycotic (*Microsporum* and *Trichophyton*), parasitic (*Demodex* and scabies), leishmanial, hormonal, and immune-mediated conditions.
iii. There is a clinical association between hypothyroidism and KCS. An estimated 20% of dogs with hypothyroidism have KCS. The blepharitis seen in this patient is in a pattern often associated with hypothyroidism, as well as the truncal alopecia, weight gain, and dry skin. A thyroid panel looking at T3, T4, thyroid-stimulating hormone, and free T4 would aid the diagnosis. A current internal medicine text will help with the details of diagnosis and treatment.

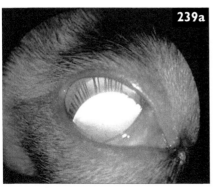 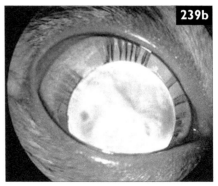

239 A five-month-old Siamese cat is presented for vaccinations.
i. Describe the lesions (239a, b). (The pupil is pharmacologically dilated.)
ii. What is the diagnosis?
iii. Does this animal possibly have a breed predisposition to this condition?
iv. What are the treatment options?

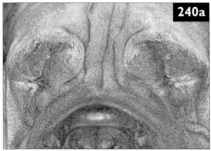 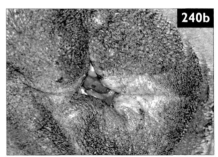

240 An adult male Mastiff was presented with severe bilateral eyelid disease and blepharospasm (240a, b).
i. Describe the clinical abnormalities noted in these photographs.
ii. What degree of entropion is present? Mild, moderate, or severe?
iii. What are some factors that may contribute to the presence and severity of the eyelid problems in this dog?
iv. What simple test that can be done to help determine if the eyelid problem present is primary (congenital or developmental) or secondary (acquired due to severe pain)?
v. What is the treatment for this condition?

239 i. The lens is small and the ciliary processes are stretched and elongated. There is a focal cataract laterally.
ii. Bilateral microphakia. The lens is smaller in volume than normal, with the result that the ciliary processes can be visualized.
iii. Siamese cats are predisposed to this congenital lens condition, but it has also been reported in domestic shorthaired cats.
iv. There is no treatment for microphakia. Patients should be monitored for lens subluxation and luxation, as well as glaucoma. (See cases **34** and **81** for presentation and treatment of lens luxations and glaucoma.)

240 i. There is bilateral lichenification, depigmentation, and hyperkeratosis of the upper and lower eyelids. Entropion is present as no normal eyelid margin can be visualized in either eye. In both eyes only a small opening allows for visualization of the globe. In **240b** a small section of visible conjunctiva is hyperemic.
ii. This Mastiff has severe entropion defined by a rolling inward of the eyelid margin of about 180 degrees. Mild entropion is a rolling inward of about 45 degrees, while moderate is about a 90 degrees rolling inward of the lid margin.
iii. Entropion can be influenced by bone structure of the orbit, skull conformation, orbital fissure length, stage of growth, excessive facial skin and folding, and gender.
iv. Topical anesthetic can be applied to the corneal surface to help differentiate between primary or anatomic entropion and secondary or spastic entropion. Careful observation is necessary after the application of the topical anesthetic.
v. Surgical repair. In this dog, multiple blepharoplastic techniques or a combination of several techniques may be necessary to correct the defects.

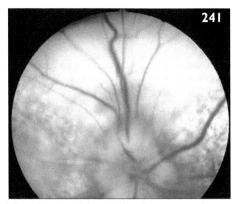

241 A five-year-old female mixed breed dog has acute glaucoma in her right eye. This image is of the right fundus (241).
i. Describe the clinical findings shown in 241.
ii. What are some possible differential diagnoses that one could make from this image?
iii. In glaucomatous dogs, what are the optic disk changes noted with regard to retinal ganglion cell death and axon loss?
iv. What ophthalmoscopic findings can be found when using the red-free filter on the direct ophthalmoscope in a dog with glaucomatous retinal and optic nerve damage?

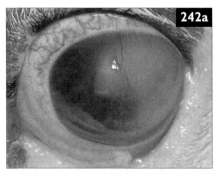 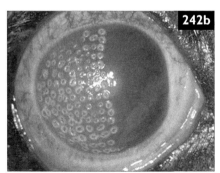

242 A seven-year-old female Boston Terrier is presented with a six-month history of increased blueness of both eyes, intraocular pressure of 18 mmHg in both eyes, and superficial nonhealing ulcers in both eyes (242a).
i. What is your diagnosis?
ii. What procedure has been performed in 242b?

241 i. Swelling of the entire optic disk is present. There are indistinct borders of the optic disk, especially from nine to three o'clock. The vessels associated with the peripheral optic disk are elevated anteriorly from retinal edema. The retina is edematous from 10 to two o'clock, as well as a focal area more peripheral to the disk at the nine o'clock position.
ii. Glaucoma and optic neuritis.
iii. The optic nerve head cup size increases in diameter and the neuroretinal rim area decreases (see case **123**). Papilledema and hemorrhage of the disk may also be noted.
iv. Dark wedge defects in the retinal sheen of the attenuated nerve fiber layer are found with the red-free filter.

242 i. The signalment (middle-aged female Boston Terrier) and clinical signs (bilateral, slowly progressive, increased corneal edema, normal IOP, and superficial nonhealing ulcers) indicate endothelial dystrophy.
ii. Patients with persistent bullae formation and nonhealing corneal ulcers may benefit from a thermokeratoplasty. This procedure will cause a change in permeability of the epithelium and contraction of the superficial stromal collagen fibers to allow movement of water out of the cornea in order to reduce corneal edema. Thermokeratoplasty is performed under heavy sedation or general anesthesia. Multifocal points of low-voltage thermal cautery are applied over the exposed stroma. The resulting corneal ulcers heal quickly.

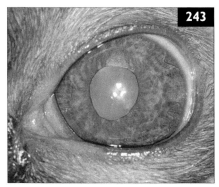

243 A nine-year-old Yorkshire Terrier was presented with an iris abnormality (243), mainly at the 12 and six o'clock positions.
i. What is the name of the condition seen in this Yorkshire Terrier?
ii. What is its etiology, and does it require treatment?

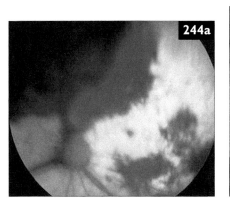

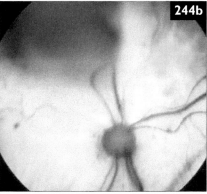

244 A 16-year-old domestic shorthaired cat was presented with acute vision loss. When questioned, the owner revealed that the cat seemed also to be polyuric and polydipsic.
i. What is the major differential for the lesions depicted in these fundus photographs (244a, b, right and left eyes, respectively)?
ii. What diagnostic tests should be performed, and what therapy can be utilized in this cat?

243 i. Senile iris atrophy (SIA).
ii. SIA is a common finding in older dogs. It is a spontaneous progressive thinning of the stroma or pupillary margin of the iris. Though it may occur in any breed, the Toy and Miniature Poodle, Miniature Schnauzer, and Chihuahua appear to have a higher incidence of this condition. The pupillary margin often develops a scalloped, moth-eaten appearance. Atrophy of the pupillary muscles results in dyscoria and may lead to reduced or absent pupillary light reflexes. Therefore, when efferent pupillary abnormalities are present, the clinician must consider iris atrophy as a possible cause. SIA may also initially manifest as a subtle fading of the natural iris color and increased pigmentation present in focal areas due to exposure of the pigmented posterior iris epithelium. As degeneration progresses, additional thinning may result in holes in the pigmented iris epithelial layers. With transillumination, affected areas appear as translucent patches or openings within the iris (as seen in 243), and are most striking when light is reflected from the tapetal fundus through the areas of affected iris. These full-thickness defects should not be mistaken for congenital iris colobomas. Vision is unaffected by iris atrophy; however, severe cases may manifest photophobia. There is no treatment for iris atrophy, although goggles and tinted contact lens have been utilized in severely photophobic dogs.

244 i. Vitreal hemorrhages and focal areas of retinal detachment are present in both eyes. The top differential is systemic hypertension. The history of polyuria/polydipsia suggests the vascular hypertension is probably secondary to renal disease. This is a common cause of acute blindness in geriatric cats (see case 159). Ocular examination may reveal retinal detachment, sub- and intraretinal hemorrhage, tortuous vessels, hyphema, vitreal hemorrhage, and glaucoma.
ii. A blood pressure reading, as well as general blood work and a urinalysis to evaluate renal function. The most common therapy to reduce the blood pressure and allow the retina to reattach is oral amlodipine (0.625 mg/cat/day).

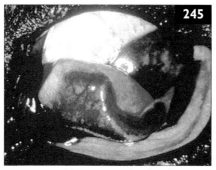

245 The left eye of a one-year-old German Shepherd Dog is shown (245).
i. What is the abnormality shown in this photo?
ii. What is the etiology?
iii. What is the treatment?

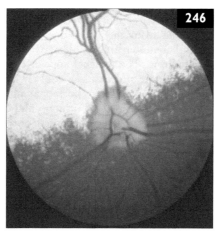

246 A dog presents with sudden blindness. Is this a normal or abnormal dog fundus image (246)?

245 i. There is an inversion of the shaft and the medial and lateral tips of the nictitating membrane (NM) cartilage.
ii. Eversion of the shaft of the NM cartilage is a commonly occurring anomaly in very large breed dogs. It may be hereditary in German Shorthaired Pointers. It is thought to result from more rapid growth of the posterior portion of the cartilage compared with that of the anterior portion. The everted cartilage appears as an anterior folding of the leading edge of the NM, with exposure of the posterior aspect. The result is chronic conjunctivitis and ocular discharge.
iii. The most popular surgical correction is excision of the folded portion of the NM cartilage. A less common anomaly of the NM cartilage (as in this case) is inversion of the medial and lateral tips of the NM cartilage. Irritation from this cartilage can result in keratitis and corneal ulceration. The bent tips can also be surgically excised if involved.

246 The fundus appears normal in both eyes this case, but the dog is blind. The diagnosis was sudden acquired retinal degeneration (SARD) based on electro-retinography (ERG) and clinical examination. SARD is a syndrome of diseases with sudden loss of vision. The differential diagnosis for sudden blindness would also include optic neuritis, cortical blindness, and retinal detachment, but there is no evidence of these conditions in this image. There are no ophthalmoscopic signs initially in SARD cases, but signs of retinal degeneration can occur weeks to months later. ERG is not detectable from the onset due to explosive photoreceptor destruction. SARD is found commonly in middle-aged, slightly obese female dogs that are also polyuric/polydipsic. The patients appear 'cushingoid'. Poodles and Dachshunds are breeds commonly affected. The etiology is unknown, but a toxic degeneration or metabolic disorder related to hormonal imbalances of melanocyte stimulating hormone or adrenocorticotropic hormone, and metabolic disturbances of the retinal pigment epithelium have been proposed. Some SARD cases may be immune mediated. Intravitreal glutamate levels are high in some cases. There is no reliable or proven therapy at present, but research continues for the etiology and treatment of SARD.

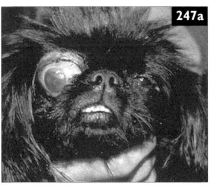
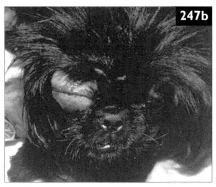

247 This adult female Pekinese (247a, b) had been diagnosed with blastomycosis and was being treated for fungal-induced anterior uveitis.
i. Describe the clinical presentation shown.
ii. What disease process causes this type of presentation?
iii. What are the treatment options for this dog?

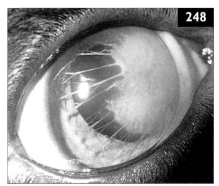
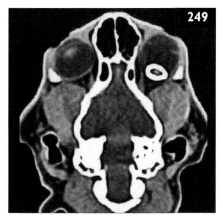

248 A 12-week-old kitten presents with a large gray spot in the center of the cornea (248).
i. Describe the lesion.
ii. What is the most likely diagnosis, and what is the etiology?
iii. What are the treatment options?

249 This is a CT image of a cat (249).
i. What are the advantages of CT scanning in veterinary ophthalmology?
ii. What ocular lesion is present?

247–249:Answers

247 i. The right globe shows moderate hyperemia of the conjunctiva, severe buphthalmia, and a swollen iris (247a).
ii. Secondary glaucoma is the most likely cause for the prominent buphthalmos. Angle obstruction from the uveitis resulted in chronic elevation in intraocular pressure (IOP). The IOP increase caused globe enlargement.
iii. The globe is severely buphthalmic and blind and it is impossible for the dog to blink completely in order to cover the cornea (247b). The globe was enucleated.

248 i. There are multiple strands of iris colored tissue extending from the iris to the cornea. The cornea has a large gray area where the strands adhere to the corneal endothelium. There is no indication of active inflammation.
ii. Persistent pupillary membranes (PPMs). In the fetus, the pupil is closed with a thin pupillary membrane that regresses prior to birth. Sometimes, regression is not complete at birth and small strands are still present until 4–5 weeks of age (see case 41). In this case the PPM is large and easily seen. PPMs are always attached to the iris collarette at one end, with the other end either floating in the anterior chamber, attached to the lens (anterior capsular cataract), attached to the iris collarette at other end, or, as in this case, adhered to the corneal endothelium, resulting in a large opacity or leukoma.
iii. The majority of PPMs require no therapy.

249 i. CT has dramatically improved the diagnosis and management of ocular and orbital disease in animals. The scanning x-ray tube of the CT machine emits a thin collimated beam of x-rays. These are attenuated as they pass through tissues and then collected by an array of special detectors. The detectors convert x-ray photons into images of thin slices of tissue (1–3 mm). The anatomy of the orbit is an ideal subject for CT. The relatively dense nerves, globe, and extraocular muscles are surrounded by lucent orbital fat and encased in dense bone and this provides a tissue of high contrast for CT. CT is used in the analysis of orbital trauma, optic neuritis, orbital infection and cellulitis, and orbital neoplasia. It can also demonstrate changes within the globe such as lens luxation, globe perforation, and intravitreal hemorrhage. Congenital optic disk colobomas can be identified, and multiple intraocular and orbital foreign bodies >0.5 mm in size can be accurately localized with CT. However, the availability of CT scanners for routine diagnostic testing is still somewhat limited and costly, and the procedure requires general anesthesia in animals.
ii. A posteriorly luxated lens is found in the eye on the right side of the image.

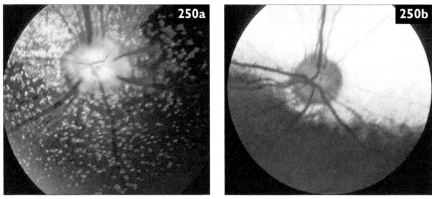

250 Two normal dog fundus images are shown (250a, b).
i. List the anatomic structures shown in these direct ophthalmoscopic images of a normal canine fundus.
ii. What is the name of the dark spot in the center of the optic nerve head (ONH)?
iii. What is the predominant cell type within the ONH?

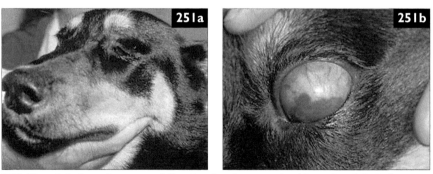

251 Enophthalmos is present following head trauma in this male adult Doberman Pinscher (251a). When the dog lowers his head the conjunctiva balloons rapidly forward (251b).
i. What is this condition, and what clinical signs are found with it?
ii. What may be the causes of this type of condition?
iii. What diagnostic tests may be performed to help confirm the condition?
iv. What is the treatment for this condition?

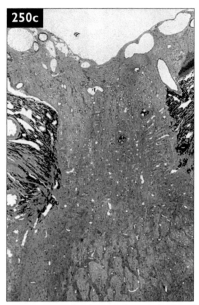

250 i. Tapetum, nontapetum, retinal vessels, and the ONH. The tapetum is granular with tapetal islets in **250a**.
ii. The physiologic pit, which is a remnant of the hyaloid artery. It is best seen in histologic specimens (**250c**, plastic section).
iii. The glial cell (the astrocyte), which provides physical support, absorbs excess extracellular potassium released by depolarizing axons, and stores glycogen.

251 i. An orbital varix, or abnormal anastomosis of orbital arteries and veins. This dog presents with an intermittent positional exophthalmos to enophthalmos that is not painful.
ii. This condition can be congenital or it can be induced by an arteriovenous anastomosis from a traumatic event, as in this dog.
iii. Diagnostic imaging such as MRI contrast studies and Doppler ultrasound can be useful.
iv. The treatment for this condition is either observation or surgical ligation of the abnormal vessels.

252 The removal of cataracts is the most common intraocular surgical procedure performed in veterinary medicine. What type of cataract removal surgery is recommended for the dog and cat?

253 The third eyelid of this kitten is attached to the dorsal conjunctiva and is not freely mobile (253). What are two possible causes for this condition?

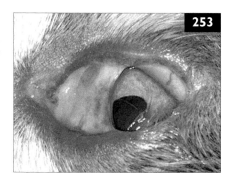

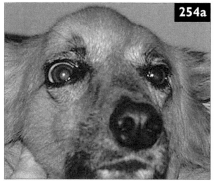

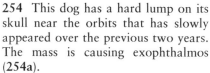

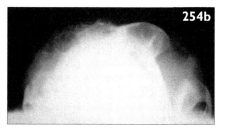

254 This dog has a hard lump on its skull near the orbits that has slowly appeared over the previous two years. The mass is causing exophthalmos (254a).
i. What is your diagnosis?
ii. How do you interpret the radiographic findings (254b, c)?

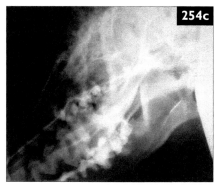

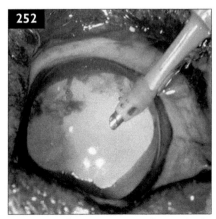

252 Phacoemulsification cataract surgery (as shown in 252) is the most useful technique for the dog and cat. This extracapsular procedure through a 3.2 mm corneal incision utilizes a piezoelectric handpiece with an ultrasonic titanium needle in a silicone sleeve to fragment and emulsify the lens nucleus and cortex following removal of the anterior capsule. The emulsified lens is then aspirated from the eye while intraocular pressure is maintained by infusion of lactated Ringer's solution or balanced salt solution. An intraocular lens implant can be inserted following cataract removal. The success rate approaches 90% for patients with healthy corneas and retinas and the absence of preoperative uveitis.

253 Abnormal adherence of conjunctiva to conjunctiva is termed symblepharon. Symblepharon is commonly associated with feline herpesvirus infections (see case 167). Symblepharon can also be due to a congenital malformation of the third eyelid, which is likely the cause in this kitten.

254 i. Neoplasia, most likely osteosarcoma, of the skull and orbit.
ii. The radiographs indicate extensive bone lysis. Multilobular osteochondro-sarcoma and osteosarcoma are other bony tumors reported in the skull of dogs; osteosarcomas of the skull are found in cats. Despite the aggressive bone lysis detected radiographically, this dog's lesion grew slowly and seemed to have limited metastatic potential over the next four years. CT and MRI can aid the diagnosis and management of skull masses.

Index

9781840761450